Health Care

OPPOSING VIEWPOINTS®

Karen Balkin, *Book Editor*

Daniel Leone, *President*
Bonnie Szumski, *Publisher*
Scott Barbour, *Managing Editor*
Helen Cothran, *Senior Editor*

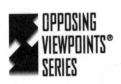

OPPOSING
VIEWPOINTS®
SERIES

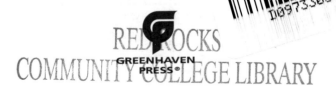

GREENHAVEN
PRESS®

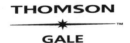

THOMSON
━━━━━✳━━━━━ ™
GALE

San Diego • Detroit • New York • San Francisco • Cleveland
New Haven, Conn. • Waterville, Maine • London • Munich

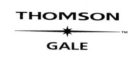

THOMSON
*
™
GALE

© 2003 by Greenhaven Press. Greenhaven Press is an imprint of The Gale Group, Inc., a division of Thomson Learning, Inc.

Greenhaven® and Thomson Learning™ are trademarks used herein under license.

For more information, contact
Greenhaven Press
27500 Drake Rd.
Farmington Hills, MI 48331-3535
Or you can visit our Internet site at http://www.gale.com

Cover credit: Creatas

LIBRARY OF CONGRESS CATALOGING-IN-PUBLICATION DATA

Health care : opposing viewpoints / Karen Balkin, book editor.
    p. cm. — (Opposing viewpoints series)
    Includes bibliographical references and index.
    ISBN 0-7377-1685-1 (lib. bdg. : alk. paper) —
    ISBN 0-7377-1686-X (pbk. : alk. paper)
    1. Medical care—United States. I. Balkin, Karen. II. Opposing viewpoints series (Unnumbered)
    RA395.A3H4123 2003
    362.1'0973—dc21
                                                                    2002041627

Printed in the United States of America

"Congress shall make no law... abridging the freedom of speech, or of the press."

First Amendment to the U.S. Constitution

The basic foundation of our democracy is the First Amendment guarantee of freedom of expression. The Opposing Viewpoints Series is dedicated to the concept of this basic freedom and the idea that it is more important to practice it than to enshrine it.

Contents

Why Consider Opposing Viewpoints?   7

Introduction   10

**Chapter 1: Is America's Health Care System in
Need of Reform?**

Chapter Preface   14

1. America Has the Best Health Care System in the
   World   16
   Joseph A. Califano Jr.

2. America Does Not Have the Best Health Care
   System in the World   23
   Bureau of Labor Education at the University of Maine

3. The Problem of Uninsured Americans Is Serious   33
   Lisa Climan and Adria Scharf

4. The Problem of Uninsured Americans Is Not
   Serious   38
   Tom Miller

5. Health Care Spending Is a Serious Problem   47
   Mick L. Diede and Richard Liliedahl

6. Health Care Spending Is Not a Serious Problem   56
   Charles R. Morris

Periodical Bibliography   66

**Chapter 2: How Has Managed Care Affected the
Health Care System?**

Chapter Preface   68

1. Managed Care Has Harmed the Health Care
   System   70
   Edmund D. Pellegrino

2. Managed Care Has Helped the Health Care
   System   79
   Gregg Easterbrook

3. Managed Care Is Necessary to Control Health
   Care Costs   89
   Thomas W. Hazlett

4. Managed Care Is Not Necessary to Control
   Health Care Costs   93
   Larry Van Heerden

5. Most Patients Are Satisfied with Managed Care   100
   Karlyn Bowman

6. Most Patients Are Not Satisfied with Managed
   Care   105
   Andrew Phillips

Periodical Bibliography   110

**Chapter 3: How Can the Problem of Uninsured
Americans Be Solved?**

Chapter Preface   112

1. Universal Health Care Is the Best Solution for
   Uninsured Americans   114
   Robert L. Ferrer

2. Universal Health Care Is Not the Best Solution
   for the Uninsured   121
   L. Dean Forman

3. Tax Credits Should Be Used to Expand Health
   Insurance Coverage   127
   Jeff Lemieux

4. Tax Credits Should Not Be Used to Expand
   Health Insurance Coverage   132
   Tom Miller

5. An Employer-Based Solution Is the Best Answer
   for the Uninsured   138
   Harry M.J. Kraemer Jr.

6. Reforming Health Care Financing Is the Best
   Answer for the Uninsured   147
   Sara J. Singer

7. Medical Savings Accounts Are the Best Answer
   for the Uninsured   154
   J. Patrick Rooney, interviewed by Jerry Geisel

Periodical Bibliography   162

Chapter 4: How Should the United States Reform Its Health Care System?

Chapter Preface	164
1. Medical IDs Would Improve the Health Care System *David Orentlicher*	166
2. Medical IDs Would Not Improve the Health Care System *Maggie Scarf*	173
3. Patients Should Be Allowed to Sue Their Health Plans *William B. Schwartz*	180
4. Patients Should Not Be Allowed to Sue Their Health Plans *Richard A. Epstein*	184
5. Physicians Should Be Allowed to Unionize *Glenn Flores*	189
6. Physicians Should Not Be Allowed to Unionize *Joshua M. Sharfstein*	193
7. Medicare Benefits Should Be Expanded to Cover Prescription Drugs *Patricia Barry*	198
8. Medicare Benefits Should Not Be Expanded to Cover Prescription Drugs *Bruce Bartlett*	204
Periodical Bibliography	208
Glossary	209
For Further Discussion	211
Organizations to Contact	213
Bibliography of Books	217
Index	219

Why Consider Opposing Viewpoints?

"The only way in which a human being can make some approach to knowing the whole of a subject is by hearing what can be said about it by persons of every variety of opinion and studying all modes in which it can be looked at by every character of mind. No wise man ever acquired his wisdom in any mode but this."

John Stuart Mill

In our media-intensive culture it is not difficult to find differing opinions. Thousands of newspapers and magazines and dozens of radio and television talk shows resound with differing points of view. The difficulty lies in deciding which opinion to agree with and which "experts" seem the most credible. The more inundated we become with differing opinions and claims, the more essential it is to hone critical reading and thinking skills to evaluate these ideas. Opposing Viewpoints books address this problem directly by presenting stimulating debates that can be used to enhance and teach these skills. The varied opinions contained in each book examine many different aspects of a single issue. While examining these conveniently edited opposing views, readers can develop critical thinking skills such as the ability to compare and contrast authors' credibility, facts, argumentation styles, use of persuasive techniques, and other stylistic tools. In short, the Opposing Viewpoints Series is an ideal way to attain the higher-level thinking and reading skills so essential in a culture of diverse and contradictory opinions.

In addition to providing a tool for critical thinking, Opposing Viewpoints books challenge readers to question their own strongly held opinions and assumptions. Most people form their opinions on the basis of upbringing, peer pressure, and personal, cultural, or professional bias. By reading carefully balanced opposing views, readers must directly confront new ideas as well as the opinions of those with whom they disagree. This is not to simplistically argue that everyone who reads opposing views will—or should— change his or her opinion. Instead, the series enhances readers' understanding of their own views by encouraging confrontation with opposing ideas. Careful examination of others' views can lead to the readers' understanding of the logical inconsistencies in their own opinions, perspective on why they hold an opinion, and the consideration of the possibility that their opinion requires further evaluation.

Evaluating Other Opinions

To ensure that this type of examination occurs, Opposing Viewpoints books present all types of opinions. Prominent spokespeople on different sides of each issue as well as well-known professionals from many disciplines challenge the reader. An additional goal of the series is to provide a forum for other, less known, or even unpopular viewpoints. The opinion of an ordinary person who has had to make the decision to cut off life support from a terminally ill relative, for example, may be just as valuable and provide just as much insight as a medical ethicist's professional opinion. The editors have two additional purposes in including these less known views. One, the editors encourage readers to respect others' opinions—even when not enhanced by professional credibility. It is only by reading or listening to and objectively evaluating others' ideas that one can determine whether they are worthy of consideration. Two, the inclusion of such viewpoints encourages the important critical thinking skill of objectively evaluating an author's credentials and bias. This evaluation will illuminate an author's reasons for taking a particular stance on an issue and will aid in readers' evaluation of the author's ideas.

It is our hope that these books will give readers a deeper understanding of the issues debated and an appreciation of the complexity of even seemingly simple issues when good and honest people disagree. This awareness is particularly important in a democratic society such as ours in which people enter into public debate to determine the common good. Those with whom one disagrees should not be regarded as enemies but rather as people whose views deserve careful examination and may shed light on one's own.

Thomas Jefferson once said that "difference of opinion leads to inquiry, and inquiry to truth." Jefferson, a broadly educated man, argued that "if a nation expects to be ignorant and free . . . it expects what never was and never will be." As individuals and as a nation, it is imperative that we consider the opinions of others and examine them with skill and discernment. The Opposing Viewpoints Series is intended to help readers achieve this goal.

David L. Bender and Bruno Leone,
Founders

Greenhaven Press anthologies primarily consist of previously published material taken from a variety of sources, including periodicals, books, scholarly journals, newspapers, government documents, and position papers from private and public organizations. These original sources are often edited for length and to ensure their accessibility for a young adult audience. The anthology editors also change the original titles of these works in order to clearly present the main thesis of each viewpoint and to explicitly indicate the opinion presented in the viewpoint. These alterations are made in consideration of both the reading and comprehension levels of a young adult audience. Every effort is made to ensure that Greenhaven Press accurately reflects the original intent of the authors included in this anthology.

Introduction

"[Medicare] will take its place beside Social Security and together they will form the twin pillars of protection upon which all our people can safely build their lives and their hopes."

—*Lyndon Johnson*

No exploration of the nation's health care system is complete without a discussion of Medicare and the principles of government-sponsored health care it represents. The concept of national health insurance for Americans was formulated almost a century ago. It was mentioned in a speech given by Louis D. Brandeis (who later became a Supreme Court justice) in 1911. It was part of former president Theodore Roosevelt's Progressive Party platform in 1912, and it was the primary agenda of the First American Conference on Social Insurance held in Chicago in 1913. Further, formal debate began in the Senate on a "standard" (universal) health insurance bill in 1915. The legislative wrangling lasted nearly fifty years, but ultimately Medicare was born.

On July 30, 1965, then-president Lyndon Johnson signed Title XVIII and Title XIX of the Social Security Act into law, making Medicare and Medicaid social and fiscal realities. Medicare provided health insurance for every American sixty-five or older. Medicaid authorized matching federal funds so that states could give additional health coverage to many elderly, low-income, and disabled people. It had taken almost half a century and the tenacious political efforts of four presidents and countless members of Congress to bring America to the point where it could offer health care insurance to its elderly population. Former president Harry Truman, a tireless advocate of government-sponsored health insurance during his administration, was present at the signing of the Medicare and Medicaid bills. Disappointed that his term in office ended before he could enact the health care legislation he knew the country needed, Truman had once written, "I have had some bitter disappointments as president, but the one that has troubled me most, in a personal way, has been the failure to defeat the organized opposition to a national compulsory health insurance program. But this opposition has only delayed and cannot stop the adoption of an indispensable federal health insurance plan."

Two issues had been key in the debate over Medicare: (1) did the aged, or a substantial number of them, need help with their medical costs? and (2) if they did, what was the best way to help them? Ultimately, Medicare critics and supporters agreed that help was needed, although they differed in their estimation of the seriousness of the problem. The primary issue, then, became the best way to provide elderly Americans with the help they needed to pay their medical bills. Three basic approaches, either separately or in combination, were considered during the original debate: (1) government subsidies for private insurance carriers, (2) direct government payments for medical services to low-income elderly through state welfare agencies, and (3) health insurance financed and administered completely through the Social Security program already in place. (The Social Security Act, minus health insurance, was signed into law on August 14, 1935.) Ultimately, legislators chose the third option, and Medicare became part of American life.

The importance of health care for the elderly has only increased as the U.S. population ages. In 1950 there were about 12 million Americans (about 8.1 percent of the population) over 65; by 1963 that number had swelled to 17.5 million (9.4 percent of the population). When Medicare became law in 1965, 19 million elderly Americans enrolled. By 2000, nearly 40 million people, almost 14 percent of the population, depended upon Medicare for health insurance coverage. As baby boomers age, the number of Medicare beneficiaries is expected to increase by at least 2 percent a year until 2015.

The steadily increasing elderly population and growing health care costs have made Medicare a more important and more complex piece of the American health care puzzle. Moreover, the time that the typical American receives Medicare benefits has increased: Nearly three years have been added to the life expectancy of the average American since Medicare began. Credit for the increase goes, in part, to expanded access to health care provided by Medicare and technological advances financed by Medicare payments. Because of Medicare's growing fiscal impact on America's economy, pressure for Medicare reform began to build in the 1990s. Some reform measures currently being debated include the option not to participate in Medicare coverage at all, barriers to fraud, formulas for reducing waste and abuse, and the addition of prescription drug benefits.

Some politicians and health care experts argue that the passage of Medicare in 1965 was as far as the United States will ever—and should ever—go in the direction of government-sponsored health insurance. They argue that an individual's medical care is too private to be overseen by the federal government. Others contend that while it has some shortcomings, the overall success of Medicare is proof that further expansion of the program into universal health care coverage is the most viable solution for the problem of uninsured Americans. More than 40 million people without health care coverage, most of them working at low-paying jobs where health care insurance is either not offered by their employers or is too expensive to purchase, have limited or no access to necessary health care.

There is no doubt that as the nation's population ages, Medicare will play an increasingly important role in the health care system. Many see the expansion of Medicare as the future of U.S. health care, ultimately leading to universal coverage and an end to what has emerged as a major health care issue of the twenty-first century—the problem of uninsured Americans. Other experts argue that Medicare must remain strong and solvent as a safety net for seniors only—it must never evolve into a system of national health care in which the government rations medical services. Medicare, universal coverage, and uninsured Americans are just a few of the issues the authors in *Health Care: Opposing Viewpoints* debate in the following chapters: Is America's Health Care System in Need of Reform? How Has Managed Care Affected the Health Care System? How Can the Problem of Uninsured Americans Be Solved? How Should the United States Reform Its Health Care System? The debate over Medicare that began almost a century ago is far from over. The issues have changed, but the purpose—to provide Americans with quality health care coverage—has not.

CHAPTER 1

Is America's Health Care System in Need of Reform?

Chapter Preface

Television and print advertising, once confined to touting over-the-counter (OTC) remedies for coughs, colds, headaches, and hemorrhoids, now tempt consumers with the latest cures—available by prescription only—for migraines, depression, high cholesterol, arthritis, asthma, and allergies. The result of these ads is that the prescription decisions that doctors used to make for their patients are now being made by patients themselves, who request (or even demand) certain drugs by name from their doctors. Some analysts argue that patients have been brainwashed into self-diagnoses by slick advertising campaigns that drive up the cost of drugs, while others maintain that intelligent health care buyers are now empowered by knowledge previously unavailable to them. Whether it is a communications innovation that is helping to improve America's health care system or an advertising mutation that demands reform, the direct-to-consumer (DTC) marketing of prescription drugs has had a profound effect on the American health care system.

Prior to the mid-1980s, drug manufacturers marketed their products only to doctors. The growth of managed care through the late 1980s and 1990s put previously unknown restrictions on the physician's prescription pad—now HMOs had a say in what drugs to prescribe—and drug marketing strategies changed. Doctors were no longer the only prescription decision-makers, so drug manufacturers began advertising directly to the group that could put the most pressure on doctors to prescribe particular drugs—consumers.

While figures differ slightly—depending on whether the source is the pharmaceutical industry or a consumer watchdog group—direct-to-consumer drug advertising topped $1.3 billion in 1997, rose to $2.5 billion in 2001, and is projected to skyrocket to $7.5 billion by 2005. Critics of DTC advertising claim that it is responsible, in great part, for the doubling of prescription drug costs between 1990 and 1997, the 17 percent increase in 1998, and 17.4 percent jump in 2000. Columnist Ellen Goodman argues, "Pharmaceutical companies tell us that the cost is connected to research and development (R&D). . . . But major drug companies, as a Families USA report shows, spend more on marketing, advertising, and administering than on R & D." Further, critics argue, DTC advertising encourages the potentially dangerous practice of self-diagnosis, where the patient decides what is wrong with him or her and the best medicine to treat the problem. A 2001 Kaiser Family Foundation survey indicated that about 44 percent of doctors do, in fact, give prescriptions for the drugs their patients request. This same survey reported that about 30 percent of television viewers requested a prescription from their doctors for a drug they saw advertised.

However, proponents of DTC advertising maintain that when patients see their symptoms in ads, they are prompted to seek help for previously undiagnosed conditions. Armed with information from ads, patients are better able to discuss their conditions with their doctors and understand the diagnoses and treatment plans. Further, business and marketing experts argue that while prescription drug costs have increased, marketing alone is not to blame. The development of new products, an aging population requiring more medication, changes in medical practices that encourage early diagnosis, preventative treatments, and disease management have all contributed to rising drug costs. According to these experts, drug manufacturers advertise their products to inform the buying public—doctors as well as patients—of a drug's effectiveness. Manufacturers would be unable to communicate the necessary information to make their drugs saleable without DTC advertising. William L. Anderson, assistant professor of business management at Frostberg State University in Maryland, contends, "Marketing doesn't drive up the price of a drug; rather, the prospect of a drug's benefits (hence, it's profitability) makes its marketing valuable."

Direct-to-consumer advertising of prescription drugs has had a significant impact on the American health care system. While some commentators argue that DTC advertising has further damaged America's health care system and made more urgent calls for reform, others contend that DTC advertising has helped change the health care system for the good. Authors in the following chapter debate the best ways to reform the nation's health care system.

"*It is imperative that the actions we take to deal with our concerns about the high cost of medical care not destroy the finest health system in the world.*"

America Has the Best Health Care System in the World

Joseph A. Califano Jr.

In the following viewpoint, Joseph A. Califano Jr. contends that the Food and Drug Administration, Public Health Service, and numerous private corporations have made the U.S. health care system great. In addition, he applauds the devoted scientists, doctors, and nurses who spend their lives in the service of others. But, he warns, aggressive managed-care reforms threaten the character and quality of American health care. Califano argues that doctors, politicians, insurers, and patients have a responsibility to safeguard the integrity of American health care. Joseph A. Califano Jr. is chairman of the National Center on Addiction and Substance Abuse at Columbia University and is a former U.S. secretary of health, education, and welfare.

As you read, consider the following questions:

1. In Califano's opinion, who was responsible for exposing the false claims and poor practices of U. S. medical schools?
2. After World War II, which government agency took over military research, according to the author?
3. What does Califano say should be required of older Americans who fail to get a free flu shot and become ill with the flu?

Joseph A. Califano Jr., "Healthy Horizons," *The American Legion Magazine*, September 1997. Copyright © 1997 by *The American Legion Magazine*. Reproduced by permission.

There is a wise old African proverb from the Bassuto tribe that Robert Ruark appropriated for his book on the Mau Mau uprisings of the 1950s: Do not destroy something of value unless you have something of value to replace it.

The United States Has the Finest System for Treating Illness and Injures

That proverb should be a warning signal and guiding principle for those who have set about the delicate task of changing America's health-care system. With all the sound and fury about the state of health care in America, too many politicians, corporate financial officers and academic economists tend to forget the most basic truth about medical care in America: We have the finest system for treating illnesses and injuries in the world. American physicians, hospitals, research centers and medical schools are the envy of the world. Heads of state and foreigners with the unlimited wealth to pay any price for the best care available flock to the United States when they are sick.

The 1990s have been marked by a headlong rush for efficiency in delivering treatment to sick and injured Americans; recognition by the for-profit sector of the big bucks to be made in taking care of what ails us; determination by the federal government to trim back funds spent on Medicare, Medicaid and other health programs for research and training if that is what it takes to balance the budget; aggressive actions by downsizing corporations to reduce costs of providing health-care benefits to employees; and increased pressures on pharmaceutical companies to reduce the price of their products even if that means forcing them to cut back on applied research.

Early Reforms Were the Beginning of Today's Greatness

Taken separately, something can be said for variations of each of these trends. Taken together, they threaten the world-class greatness that has characterized America's medical-treatment system for most of this century.

It's time for each of us to look at what made America's health-care system the finest in the world and demand that those who would dramatically restructure it count to 10 before they lose sight of the conditions that made our system great.

What makes America's health-care system great is its ability to attract the finest minds in our society to devote their lives to caring for the ill and to conducting research to attack seemingly intractable medical problems. Also critical to the special quality of care here is the commitment of doctors and nurses to health care as a ministry; not an industry. It wasn't always this way.

At the end of the 19th century and into the early years of the 20th century, American medicine was crowded with charlatans and hustlers. Doctors were poorly trained. Many medical schools were as wacky in what they taught as a Three Stooges movie. Traveling salesmen hawked potions laced with cocaine that hooked thousands of Midwest housewives who thought they were buying relief for everything from arthritis and menstrual cramps to depression and heart disease.

Then, in 1910, Abraham Flexner exposed the false claims, shoddy curriculum, facilities and faculties of many medical schools. Shocked into action by the public outcry and supported by the good physicians, states passed laws instituting stiff licensing requirements and high standards for doctors and the medical schools that trained them.

About this time, states also enacted statutes severely restricting the practice of medicine to licensed physicians, and Congress established the Food and Drug Administration and gave it the power to test medications to make certain they were safe and effective before they could be marketed to Americans.

As a result of these actions, the quality of medical education and physicians soared. Doctors whose average 19th century income put them in the lower middle class, rose rapidly in economic and social status in their communities. The words, "my son the doctor," became the prayer and dream of a generation of immigrants. And the best and the brightest men and women were attracted to the medical profession.

Over time, thanks to the system of clearing pharmaceuticals by the FDA, this nation avoided tragedies that beset other countries. In Britain, for example, thousands of children were born deformed as a result of mothers taking thalidomide. We avoided that situation—and others like it—here because of the tough review requirements to which drugs were subjected before they could be prescribed by physicians or sold over the counter. More than any other people in the world, Americans could be confident that the medicine they were given would work and that those medicines would be safe to take.

America Is a Leader in Medical Research

Since World War II, government-funded research has sparked a stunning record of scientific and medical advances. The development of vaccines and their translation into the daily practice of medicine have helped reduce the incidence of, and in some cases eradicate, diseases such as smallpox, hepatitis B virus, measles, and polio. New treatments have been developed to treat cancer, heart disease, and mental illness. Increases in life expectancy and improvements in health drastically improved living standards in the United States as well as the nation's economic health. . . .

The new millennium promises even greater advances. The government-supported Human Genome Project has revolutionized the understanding of the basic building blocks of life, as well as the structure and causes of disease. With the sequencing of the genome, genetic tests will soon be accurate predictors of the risk of disease, and interventions may be targeted to effectively prevent and treat numerous diseases.

William H. Frist, "Federal Funding for Biomedical Research: Commitment and Benefits," *Journal of the American Medical Association*, April 3, 2002.

In the earliest days of the Republic—1789—we established a Public Health Service. At the turn of the 20th century, Congress began expanding the mission of the Public Health Service to include the study of infectious diseases and control of epidemics. But the role of the national government in public health and biomedical research was marginal up to World War II.

As part of the nation's mobilization for World War II, the federal government made substantial investments in public health, training professionals and medical research. The armed forces needed physicians and nurses, so they drafted all they could get their hands on and trained even more. Medical research was conducted on everything from frostbite to malaria, from venereal disease to surgical and burn procedures. Public health programs were mounted to protect soldiers from sexually transmitted diseases and keep production workers on the home front healthy and strong. Wonder drugs like penicillin, new surgical procedures for wounds and burns and prosthetic devices to replace lost limbs were developed.

At the end of the war, the military research effort was transferred to the National Institutes of Health. In the postwar years, these institutes became the central workhorse for basic biomedical research. Sparked by the bipartisan commitment of Presidents Lyndon Johnson and Richard Nixon, who declared billion-dollar-a-year wars on cancer and cardiovascular disease, the National Institutes of Health and the National Cancer Institute became the finest basic biomedical research operation in the world. The brightest scientists in the United States and many foreign nations competed either to work there or to receive grants to work at research centers throughout the nation.

In the 1940s and 1950s most large corporations started including health insurance coverage as part of their basic wage and benefits package, and the government built half a million hospital beds. In the 1960s, with President Johnson calling upon Americans to create a Great Society, Congress passed Medicare to provide physician and hospital care for all citizens 65 and older and Medicaid to provide such care to the poor and nursing home care to the elderly who needed it. Congress enacted heart, cancer and stroke legislation and American citizens no longer had to travel to New York or Boston for the finest health care. It would now be available in world-class medical centers across the country, from Seattle to Miami, Los Angeles and Houston to Philadelphia, New Orleans and Chicago.

Quality and Trust Must Not Be Sacrificed to Save Money

It is imperative that the actions we take to deal with our concerns about the high cost of medical care not destroy the finest health system in the world. It is important to deliver medical diagnosis and treatment at the lowest possible cost.

But we must not let our infatuation with managed-care organizations—using the profit motive to make treatment more efficient, downsizing corporations and cutting federal and state budgets—destroy what is good in American health care. For at its best, medical treatment in the United States has no peer.

Managed-care plans are double-edged swords. The smooth edge can cut costs in the delivery of treatment. But the jagged edge can increase bureaucracy and tear at quality, trust and the human touch that have been the defining marks of American health care. Due largely to managed care, in 1997 Americans will spend $200 billion for the paperwork of submitting, reviewing, approving, billing and paying claims. Doctors and nurses must now be masters of the universe of bureaucratic haggling and manipulation as well as masters of medicine.

The pressure for efficiency also leaves physicians little time to talk to patients. If a managed-care physician has 15 minutes to see a patient, what happens at the end of an exam when the patient says to him that her husband is beating her or someone tells him that he's impotent. Medical advice at that point does not fit into a few minutes. We should insist that in the quest for efficiency, we pay doctors for the time they spend talking to patients.

Patients Must Always Come First

Patients, doctors, employers and insurers can all take steps to avert the danger of a decline of quality and trust between doctors and patients. If your doctor doesn't have time to talk to you, fire him and get one who will. Doctors should resist attempts to put profits above patients and efforts to interfere with the doctor-patient relationship or the exercise of their best medical judgment. Employers should provide avenues through which their employees and retirees can complain about reductions in quality of care.

As citizens, we should also keep close tabs on the politicians who want to cut investments in basic biomedical research and support for medical education. We didn't get so many of our best minds into research on cardiovascular disease, cancer, arthritis and AIDS by waving a magic wand.

They were attracted by the national, bipartisan commitment to support basic biomedical research and our willingness to recognize the importance of providing reasonable profits to pharmaceutical companies to encourage their investment in applied research to produce, distribute and educate the medical professions about miracle drugs, diagnostic procedures and medical devices.

We should recognize that Medicare is a phenomenal success at providing health care to elderly Americans. There is room for improvement and efficiencies. We can take steps to encourage older Americans to take better care of themselves. For example, Medicare provides free flu vaccinations. Less than 40 percent of eligible individuals take advantage of this Medicare benefit. Why not require those who become ill because they failed to get a flu shot pay the medical expenses for their treatment? Since Medicare beneficiaries who smoke need more medical care than those who don't, why not charge the smokers higher premiums? It might encourage them to quit. It makes more sense to take actions to encourage the elderly to take better care of themselves than to cut the benefits available to them when they get sick.

Medicine Is Not an Industry

Most importantly, let each of us insist that our politicians, corporate executives and for-profit health companies accept and act on these fundamental truths: Medicine is a sacred ministry, not an industry. Touching will always be a part of healing. The highest calling of doctors and nurses is to protect and preserve life, heal the sick and comfort the dying. Each of us has a responsibility to pursue healthy lifestyles. If all the actors in the system of American health care live by these basic values, then we can be certain that our grandchildren will live in a nation whose medical treatment remains the envy of the rest of the world.

"As its major shortcomings become more visible, Americans are finding it harder to accept [the assertion that the United States has the best health care system in the world]."

America Does Not Have the Best Health Care System in the World

Bureau of Labor Education at the University of Maine

In the following viewpoint, the Bureau of Labor Education at the University of Maine argues that America's low ranking on a 2000 World Health Organization (WHO) survey highlights the problems that plague the American health care system. According to the bureau, while the United States spends the most on health care of any developed country, it ranks far below the others in overall performance and fairness of financial contributions. A single payer plan might give Americans the health care they are already paying for but not getting, the bureau maintains. The bureau is part of the University of Maine's Division of Lifelong Learning and provides research and education to Maine workers.

As you read, consider the following questions:

1. According to this viewpoint, what did WHO establish as the three primary goals of a good health care system?
2. In which of the three primary goals does the United States rank first, according to the bureau?
3. If the United States changed to a single payer health care plan, what role does the bureau see for private insurers?

Bureau of Labor Education at the University of Maine, "The U.S. Health Care System: Best in the World, or Just the Most Expensive?" *Issues Brief*, Summer 2001, pp. 1–8. Copyright © 2001 by Bureau of Labor Education at the University of Maine. Reproduced by permission.

For many years, politicians and insurance companies could blithely proclaim that the U.S. had the best health care system in the world, but as its major shortcomings become more visible, Americans are finding it harder to accept this assertion. The 42.6 million people in the U.S. currently without health insurance are acutely aware that our health care system is not working for everyone, and there is growing recognition that the major problems of rising costs and lack of access constitute a real crisis. However, the search for solutions has not been easy or clear cut. Policymakers often attempt to address the symptoms of our health care crisis through short-term, patchwork solutions, under the pressure of time and the constraints of political decision-making, rather than analyzing the system itself as a whole. One important step in searching for effective longer-term solutions is to ask a deceptively simple two-fold question: how can we know whether a health care system is both "good"—that is, how well it does its job—and fair, in terms of financing health costs? If we can then analyze how well our health system performs, in comparison to other countries in the world, we will have a basis from which to explore possible alternatives.

Characteristics of a Good and Fair Health Care System

A number of recent studies have compared the health systems of various countries. Using information and concepts from these studies, it is possible to evaluate the health care system of the U.S. and other countries, with respect to such fundamental issues as cost, access to health care, and how well the health system succeeds in producing good health outcomes in a population.

The World Health Organization (WHO) released a groundbreaking report in 2000, with data on the health systems of 191 member countries. In this analysis, WHO developed three primary goals for what a good health system should do: 1) *good health:* "making the health status of the entire population as good as possible" across the whole life cycle, 2) *responsiveness:* responding to people's expectations of respectful treatment and client orientation by health care providers, and 3) *fairness in financing:* ensuring financial protection for everyone, with costs distributed according to one's ability to pay. The WHO study also distinguished between the overall "goodness" of health care systems ("the best attainable average level") and fairness ("the smallest feasible differences among individuals and groups"). A health system which is both good and fair would thus ideally have:

1. Overall good health (e.g., low infant mortality rates and high disability-adjusted life expectancy).

2. A fair distribution of good health (e.g., low infant mortality and long life expectancy evenly distributed across population groups).

3. A high level of overall responsiveness.

4. A fair distribution of responsiveness across population groups.

5. A fair distribution of financing health care (whether the burden of health costs is fairly distributed, based on ability to pay, so that everyone is equally protected from the financial risks of illness).

Other major sources of international health system data include the OECD (Organization for Economic Cooperation and Development) data on its 29 member countries, the U.S. Census Bureau, and other international studies, including two studies comparing patient satisfaction in various countries. By using these health system data, we can compare the U.S. with a number of other roughly comparable, high-income OECD countries (e.g., relatively developed or industrialized).

U.S. Health Care Is the Most Costly

Here are some basic facts that stand out in doing such international comparisons:

Cost: The United States has by far the most expensive health care system in the world, based on health expenditures per capita (per person), and on total expenditures as a percentage of gross domestic product (GDP). As shown in Figure One and Table One, the United States spent $4,178 per capita on health care in 1998, more than twice the OECD median of $1,783, and far more than its closest competitor, Switzerland ($2,794). U.S. health spending as a percentage of GDP, 13.6 percent in 1998, also outdistanced the next most expensive health systems, in Germany (10.6 percent) and Switzerland (10.4 percent).

The reasons for the especially high cost of health care in the U.S. can be attributed to a number of factors, ranging from the rising costs of medical technology and prescription drugs to the high administrative costs resulting from the complex multiple payer system in the U.S. For example, it has been estimated that between 19.3 and 24.1 percent of the total dollars spent on health care in the U.S. is spent simply on administrative costs. The growing shift from non-profit to for-profit health care providers, such as the growth of for-profit hospital chains, has also contributed to the increased costs of health care. By 1994, research showed that administrative costs among for-profit hospitals had increased to *34.0 percent*, compared to 24.5 percent for private non-profit hospitals, and 22.9 percent for public hospitals.

In addition, the high proportion of people who are uninsured in the U.S. (15.5 percent in 1999) contributes to expensive health care because conditions that could be either prevented or treated inexpensively in the early stages often develop into health crises. Treatment of crisis conditions

Figure One. Health Spending Per Capita in Selected High-Income OECD Countries (in U.S. Dollars), 1998

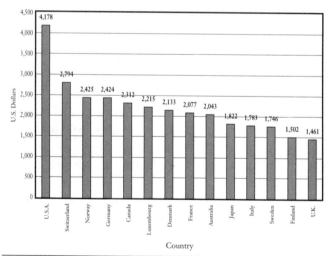

later on is much more expensive, such as emergency room treatment, or intensive care when an untreated illness progresses to a more serious stage. Finally, the aging of the population in the U.S. is also contributing to mounting increases in the cost of health care.

Given that we spend so much more of our societal resources on health care, what kind of return is the nation's population receiving? This can be addressed by looking at some measures of health outcomes.

Do Health Outcomes Justify Spending?

Access to health care: *The U.S. is "the only country in the developed world, except for South Africa, that does not provide health care for all of its citizens."* Instead, we have a confusing hodgepodge of private insurance coverage based primarily on employment, along with public insurance coverage for the elderly (Medicare), the military, veterans, and for the poor and disabled (Medicaid, which varies greatly in its implementation across states). Such a "non-system" creates serious gaps in coverage. And as insurance rates rise, more and more employers are forced to either drop their insurance benefits altogether, or to raise premiums and deductibles.

According to the most recently available figures, *42.6 million people in America were uninsured in 1999*, down slightly from 1997 and 1998 figures. It is an embarrassment to many policy makers in the U.S. that we do not have universal coverage, but more seriously, it is a matter of life and death in many cases for people who do not have access to care. As the American College of Physicans-American Society of Internal Medicine has pointed out, "people without health insurance tend to live sicker and die younger than people with health insurance." The lack of health insurance for a significant portion of Americans also has other far-reaching consequences, as hospitals and other care providers are forced into cost shifting, at the expense of taxpayers and higher premiums for those with private insurance.

Health and Well-Being: There are many different indicators of the overall health status and well-being of a country's population, but among the most commonly used measures are infant mortality rates, and life expectancy, particularly

Table One. Health Care System Indicators and Rankings in Selected High-Income OECD Countries, 1997–1999

Country	(OECD) Health Spending Per Capita in U.S. Dollars, 1998	(OECD) Health Spending as a Percent of GDP, 1998	(US Census) Infant Mortality Rate, 1998	(WHO) Disability-Adjusted Life Expectancy & Rank, 97/99	(WHO, Rank) Fairness of Financial Contributions, 1997	(WHO, Rank) Responsiveness of Health System, 1997	(WHO, Rank) Health System Overall Performance, 1997	(See Blendon) Percent Satisfied with Health System, 1998 & 2000
United States	4,178	13.6	7.2	70.0 (24)	54–55	1	37	40
Australia	2,043	8.5	5.2	73.2 (2)	26–29	12–13	32	N.A.
Canada	2,312	9.5	5.2	72.0 (12)	17–19	7–8	30	46
Denmark	2,133	8.3	5.2	69.4 (28)	3–5	4	34	91
Finland	1,502	6.9	3.9	70.5 (20)	8–11	19	31	81
France	2,077	9.6	4.6	73.1 (3)	26–29	16–17	1	65
Germany	2,424	10.6	4.9	70.4 (22)	6–7	5	25	58
Italy	1,783	8.4	6.1	72.7 (6)	45–47	22–23	2	20
Japan	1,822	7.6	4.0	74.5 (1)	8–11	6	10	N.A.
Luxembourg	2,215	5.9	5.1	71.1 (18)	2	3	16	67
Norway	2,425	8.9	4.0	71.7 (15)	8–11	7–8	11	N.A.
Sweden	1,746	8.4	3.5	73.0 (4)	12–15	10	23	58
Switzerland	2,794	10.4	4.7	72.5 (8)	38–40	2	20	N.A.
U.K.	1,461	6.7	5.9	71.7 (14)	8–11	26–27	18	57
OECD Median	1,783	8.2						

disability-adjusted life expectancy ("the number of healthy years that can be expected on average in a given population"). As of 1998, the infant mortality rate in the United States was 7.2 infant deaths per 1,000 live births (identical to the rates for 1996 and 1997). Although this number is a historic low for the U.S., our infant mortality rate is nonetheless the highest among the OECD countries in Table One and Figure Two. In 1996, *the U.S. ranked 26th among industrialized countries for infant mortality rates.*

These infant mortality figures for the U.S. are somewhat misleading, however, since they obscure the persisting wide disparities among racial groups, based in large part on economic differences. As the U.S. Department of Health and Human Services indicates, the infant mortality rate for black children (14.3 in 1998) is more than twice that of white children (6.0 deaths per 1,000 live births), and it is higher still in some areas of the country. For example, the 1999 infant mortality rate for black children in Alabama was 16.0 infant deaths before age one, among 1,000 live births. Many health policy analysts consider such figures a shocking indictment of living conditions for segments of the population in the richest country on earth.

The WHO figures also show that *the U.S. ranks very low (24th) on disability-adjusted life expectancy (DALE)* among high-income OECD countries (see Table One); only Denmark ranked lower (28th). The U.S. also has a very unequal distribution of disability-adjusted life expectancy; particularly among males (in which some segments have a much longer disability-free life expectancy than others). This should not come as a surprise, however. When a sizable portion of the population lacks access to health care, particularly preventive care, one should expect that they would also be likely to experience more years of disability.

United States Leads in Responsiveness

Responsiveness: Based on WHO's international comparisons, *the U.S. was first among the 191 member countries in the category of responsiveness*, the extent to which caregivers are responsive to client/patient expectations with regard to non-health areas such as being treated with dignity and respect,

Figure Two. Infant Mortality Rates in Selected High-Income OECD Countries, 1998

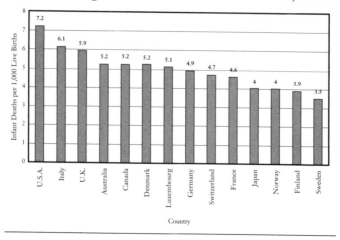

Country

etc. However, this figure almost certainly covers over the existence of extreme disparities in responsiveness among different populations. In particular, it is obvious that the millions of people with either no insurance or else very limited access to health care via Medicaid, etc., have far greater problems finding responsive caregivers than those with an adequate degree of private health insurance coverage.

Fairness in Financing: This measures the degree to which financial contributions to health systems are distributed fairly across the population. Table One shows that while OECD countries such as Luxembourg, Denmark and Germany have health systems which are very fair in financial contributions to the system, other countries such as the U.S. and Italy have very unfair systems of health financing. *The U.S was the lowest (least fair) of all the OECD countries in Table One; tied for 54th and 55th place.*

An unfair system of financing has consequences for much of the population, but especially for those who are uninsured or underinsured, and for the poor. As the WHO report states, "the impact of failures in health systems is most severe on the poor everywhere, who are driven deeper into poverty by lack of financial protection against ill-health."

Attainment and Performance: In addition to evaluating the

world's various health care systems using these criteria and providing other relevant health-related information, the WHO also ranked the world's countries in terms of the overall *attainment* of their health systems (based on all five of the criteria, above), and the *performance* of their health systems—that is, how well a country's health system is performing, compared to how well it could perform given its levels of resources. The results for overall attainment and performance were quite revealing: among the 191 countries listed, *the U.S. health care system ranked 15th in the world for overall attainment* (data not included in Table One), and *37th in the world for performance* (see Table One).

Satisfaction with Health Care System: One more interesting question is the extent to which ordinary people are satisfied with their country's health care system. As shown in Table One, the two countries with the highest percentage of people who were either very satisfied or fairly satisfied with their country's health care system overall were Denmark (91 percent!) and Finland (81 percent). Italy was the lowest among the European Union countries surveyed in the "Eurobarometer" study, at 20 percent. *The U.S. was comparatively low also, with only 40 percent of people who were satisfied* with their health care system. Even the United Kingdom, which has had persisting problems with its national health service in recent years, had almost 60 percent of its people saying they were either very satisfied or fairly satisfied.

A Single Payer Plan Could Be the Answer

This viewpoint has briefly described some of the most critical problems affecting the health care system in the U.S., such as access to health care, high costs, fairness, and effectiveness in bringing about good health in its population. There are many other major issues which also contribute to our mounting health care crisis, such as declining patient choices, the increased control in health care decisions by managed care companies as they seek to further limit access to care, the crisis in the nursing profession as nurses desert the profession in droves, and quality of care issues. It is becoming increasingly clear that these continuing dilemmas are unlikely to be solved without a thorough and creative overhaul of our present system.

Despite the efforts of insurance companies and managed care companies to limit the range of political choices in health care reforms, there appears to be growing broad-based support in the U.S. for a single payer system which would greatly resolve some of the most serious problems of cost, access and fairness. Furthermore, recent studies have shown that a single payer plan would not only be economically feasible, but would be an enormous improvement over what we have. In 1991, for example, both the U.S. General Accounting Office (GAO) and the Congressional Budgeting Office (CBO) issued reports stating that a single payer system similar to that of Canada's would more than pay for itself, due to reduced administrative costs, as well as having universal access to health care, especially preventive care. A single payer health insurance plan would not rule out a continuing role for private insurers, since it would probably provide only a basic level of coverage. In addition, recent surveys in the U.S. have documented the growing frustration with our health care system, and an interest in exploring a single payer plan for health insurance with universal coverage. Finally, recent efforts by Massachusetts health care policy analysts have shown that a single payer health care plan in Massachusetts would also be economically feasible.

One possible approach that has been advocated by some health care experts, for example, is to simply expand Medicare, an existing and highly successful public program which could be extended beyond the elderly to the entire population. Interestingly, Medicare costs for administration are currently less than two percent. This and other alternative models need to be explored and discussed, with the help of current and unbiased information. It is clearly imperative, therefore, that policymakers and lay people alike educate ourselves on the issues, and to exercise our collective imagination and creativity in meeting these challenges.

"The outlook remains bleak for those living without health coverage."

The Problem of Uninsured Americans Is Serious

Lisa Climan and Adria Scharf

In the following viewpoint, Lisa Climan and Adria Scharf tell the stories of some of the individuals who make up America's 42.5 million uninsured. The people they profile are real—they are the names behind the numbers, according to the authors. Climan and Scharf maintain that because these families can not afford coverage, they do not get the health care they need. Lack of insurance means they live with pain and worry, and assume huge debts when they do seek medical care, according to the authors. Adria Scharf is coeditor of and Lisa Climan is a contributing writer to *Dollars & Sense*.

As you read, consider the following questions:

1. According to Climan and Scharf, which country is the only industrialized nation without a sound insurance program?
2. What is the definition of "low income," according to the authors?
3. About what percentage of the uninsured are adults?

Lisa Climan and Adria Scharf, "Putting Names on the Numbers," *Dollars & Sense*, May 2001, p. 32. Copyright © 2001 by Kaiser Family Foundation. Reproduced by permission.

The United States is the only modern industrialized country without a sound health insurance program. In 1999, one in six non-elderly U.S. residents—more than 42.5 million people—went without health coverage for the entire year. During the economic boom of the 1990s, the number of uninsured actually grew, both in terms of raw numbers and in terms of their proportion of the total population.

Don't expect the situation to improve any time soon. Even with a vast budget surplus at their disposal, neither Republicans nor Democrats plan to increase public spending for social needs. Instead, they want to spend the surplus on tax cuts and paying down the national debt. Either way, the outlook remains bleak for those living without health coverage, and for recipients of Medicaid and Medicare as well.

Below are highlights from the Kaiser Commission on Medicaid and the Uninsured's new report, *In Their Own Words: The Uninsured Talk About Living Without Health Insurance*. The report profiles families who cannot afford the coverage they need. As a result, they postpone medical care, live in pain, worry, and take on crushing debt when they inevitably do seek medical attention.

The Smith Family, Paterson, New Jersey

Each time a fever struck one of her daughters during the two anxious years when they didn't have health insurance, Yolanda Smith would ask herself a series of questions: How high was the temperature? What could she do to bring it down? Was it serious enough to require a doctor's attention?

If the fever persisted, Yolanda might wait it out one more day. If it still hadn't come down, she would reluctantly borrow $40 from her mother to pay the fee that the doctor's office required up front. If her mother didn't have the money, Yolanda would play her last card and take her daughter to the emergency room, knowing that the bill for that visit, though huge, would drift in later.

Like the majority of uninsured Americans, Yolanda, 29, works full-time, in her case, as a customer service representative for a cigar-distribution company. Part of the appeal of Yolanda's new job was that it offered health insurance. But Yolanda suffered sticker shock when she found out what her share of the cost would be. To cover herself alone, she had to pay $85 every two weeks. Coverage that would include her daughters would have cost $150 every two weeks, an amount she simply could not figure out a way to pay.

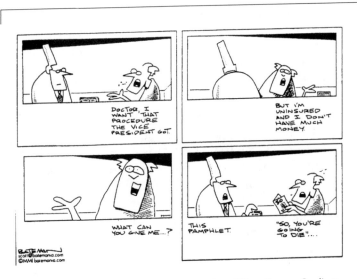

Bateman. © 2001 by MMI. Reprinted by permission of Kings Features Syndicate.

Yolanda earns $12.50 an hour, or about $26,000 a year. That puts her squarely in the hardscrabble territory of low income America, defined as those who earn less than 200% of the federal poverty level, or $28,300 for a family of three in 2000. It is these workers and their families, living just a few handholds above poverty, that run the second highest risk, after the poor, of being uninsured.

The Nelson Family, Louisville, Tennessee

Nobody needs to tell Patricia Nelson how important health insurance is. When her husband William was just 35 years old, he developed Lou Gehrig's disease. The disability-linked insurance provided by Medicare meant that in the final months of his illness, Patricia could care for him in their own home, with doctors, nurses, and therapists stopping by as needed, at little cost to the family.

Despite Patricia's understanding of the significance of insurance, she and her son Sam have been going without it since June 2000, one month after she left a job with health benefits to help a sister and brother-in-law strengthen their family business.

Like many Americans, Patricia has found over the years that her family's access to health insurance has depended largely on the decisions of employers. For 10 years, from 1983 through 1993, Patricia worked in a restaurant, making just above minimum wage. "Sometimes there was insurance, and sometimes there wasn't, depending on who the owners were," she says.

The most costly uninsured medical expense came when Sam was five years old and had a bad asthma attack. At Children's Hospital, the billing office checked on whether Sam was eligible for Medicaid. Patricia remembers the family missing the eligibility cutoff by $4. "We were in there for two days, and I ended up with a $6,000 hospital bill that I'm still paying $25 a month on," Patricia says. Her balance, after seven years of paying, is $1,790.

She prays that she and Sam stay healthy and injury-free. "The thing is, you can't get private insurance for a price you can afford," she says.

Note: After the Kaiser report was issued, Patricia Nelson lost her job when her sister's business closed down. She has since developed a serious kidney infection, and Sam now has Bell's Palsy. Faced with over $12,000 in medical bills, she has filed for bankruptcy.

The Roberts Family, Bena, Virginia

Through the years, Tom, now 46, has worked hard to provide for his family. He's worked at lots of different jobs—as an assistant minister, a sheet metal fabricator, a Hawaiian Punch can assembler, a machine mechanic, a painter, and a construction supervisor. Not all of those jobs provided him with health insurance, though. In fact, he and the family often weren't covered. They paid for health care as they needed it and put off what they could.

The Roberts don't believe they're owed anything—not by the government, not by employers. But Tom would like to see companies take more responsibility for their employees.

He remembers what it was like growing up in New Jersey, where his father, a union electrical worker, always had good employer-provided health insurance for his whole family. Tom also remembers his own experiences with employers that provided good coverage. "We were well taken care of," he recalls. But as time went on, those kind of jobs have become harder to find.

"It may be wrong on my part," he says, "but I think an employer as large as mine—a medical corporation—could do something for its employees, like my father had or like I once had."

Who Are the Uninsured?

• Most are people who work, or their dependents. Over two-thirds (71%) come from families with at least one full-time worker. Only 18% come from families where no one is employed.

• Many are not poor. Over a third (35%) come from families with incomes above 200% of the poverty line. Just under a third (29%) come from near-poor families, with incomes between 100 and 200% of the poverty line. Thirty-six percent come from families with incomes below the poverty line ($13,290 for a family of three in 1999).

• Three quarters (75%) are adults. Because of government insurance programs that target children, adults are at greater risk of being uninsured than children.

• Half of the uninsured are white, but minorities, particularly Hispanics, are at much greater risk of being uninsured than whites.

VIEWPOINT

4

*"We should reexamine the too facile
presumption that more health care is
always good, and, because it improves access
to more health care, more health insurance
coverage is always . . . desirable."*

The Problem of Uninsured
Americans Is Not Serious

Tom Miller

In the following viewpoint, originally presented as part of a
Cato Institute Policy Forum, Tom Miller argues that providing uninsured Americans health insurance won't necessarily improve their access to health care or their health.
Poor health among the uninsured, he contends, is due to factors other than lack of insurance, such as illiteracy and unhealthy lifestyle practices. Moreover, Miller maintains, lack
of insurance does not keep uninsured Americans from getting the health care they need nor does it cause them undue
financial hardship. Tom Miller is director of Health Policy
Studies at the Cato Institute.

As you read, consider the following questions:
1. According to Miller, health insurance is only of value
   when it does what three things?
2. In the author's opinion, what determines disparities in
   infant health at birth?
3. Reductions in the price of health care disproportionately
   benefit what group, according to Miller?

Tom Miller, "Will More Health Insurance Improve Health Outcomes?" *Cato
Institute Policy Forum*, June 2002. Copyright © 2002 by The Cato Institute.
Reproduced by permission.

As a general overview and warning, I would suggest you be skeptical of any and all sweeping claims about single factor explanations for what improves or impairs health status and health outcomes. In particular, we should reexamine the too facile presumption that more health care is always good, and, because it improves access to more health care, more health insurance coverage is always also desirable, if not necessary.

We need to be concerned with the appropriate measure of the bottom line by focusing on the output, not the input. Health insurance only provides value to the extent that it improves health outcomes, it improves our health status, and it protects us from serious financial risk.

Now, the assumption that health insurance affects health outcomes is a longstanding one, but also a relatively soft one. Consider that it may also be held much less due to persuasive evidence than as an act of faith, or even as a cover for self-interested parties seeking primarily to get paid more predictably and more adequately for their health services invoices. Nevertheless, we are in the midst of the latest wave of megastudies that purport to cement the connection between expanded health insurance coverage—financed by public subsidies—and improved health. The latest entrant is the study *Care Without Coverage: Too Little, Too Late*, by a committee of the Institute of Medicine (IOM). . . .

The study is the second of a series of six planned IOM studies along these lines. It aims to disabuse us of the notion that Americans without health insurance manage to get the care that they really need. It finds instead that working-age individuals without health insurance are more likely to receive too little medical care and receive it too late, be sicker and die sooner, and receive poorer care even when they're in the hospital for acute situations.

IOM Study Compares No Health Coverage to Complete Coverage

Of course, you always need a headline grabber in this field, and this study furnished the factoid that more than 18,000 adults die each year in the U.S. because they are uninsured and can't get proper health care. Now, the study appears to compare working-age people with no health coverage at all with those who have relatively complete health insurance coverage. There is no noticeable effort to compare the outcomes of the uninsured with people who may have incomplete or limited coverage, such as catastrophic coverage.

There is also an earlier Institute of Medicine study which asked whether it's possible to sort out and disentangle the effects of race, socioeconomic status and insurance coverage on health. Jennifer Haas and Nancy Adler, in October 2001, in what's called *The Causes of Vulnerability*, note that most studies have examined utilization of health care rather than health status as the outcome measure, and measures of health care utilization and process of care are more strongly and consistently influenced by insurance status than are measures of health status alone.

Other factors besides health insurance remain on the table as determinants of poor health, and they include low literacy, lifestyle practices, and health benefits. Haas and Adler find that the implementation of universal coverage in other countries may narrow disparities in health utilization but not disparities in health. Ethnic and socioeconomic disparities in health persist.

Despite mixed evidence at best, though, the paper then hurtles on to a conclusion that, given the political obstacles to other types of broad societal interventions that might attempt to reduce ethnic and socioeconomic disparities in health, health insurance may be a necessary first step toward improving health status in the U.S. In other words, why not take what the political defense gives you?

Recent Study Unclear on the Benefits of Insurance

Also out in May 2002 is a lengthy study by Jack Hadley, of the Urban Institute, for the Kaiser Family Foundation, called *Sicker and Poorer: The Consequences of Being Uninsured*. It notes that none of the many studies it reviews on the positive relationships between health insurance, use of medical care, health, income, and education is definitive, nor are their findings universal.

Hadley suggests, though, we should distinguish between

studies that suggest little or no health benefit from additional medical care use by well-insured populations and those studies suggesting that the uninsured would benefit from health insurance coverage and greater medical care use. He does not indicate how politicians and interest groups will draw that distinction and then carefully prioritize and target narrowly any future round of expanded health insurance subsidies, however. . . .

Now, within the limits of mostly observational studies in this field, Hadley provides an estimated range of the quantitative effects of extending health insurance coverage to all the uninsured, and suggests that their mortality rates would decline by at least 5 percent. One of his most promising recommendations is to develop new health insurance experiments that are drawn from a population of the currently uninsured, and then randomly assign some of them to a treatment group receiving insurance coverage. We don't have that experiment yet.

But on the health economist's other hand, sometimes including the more invisible hand of the market, a number of other studies raise many questions about the "more health insurance, better health care" connection. Not all those studies point in exactly the same direction and reach an integrated, mutually consistent set of conclusions, so a dose of humility and skepticism is in order across the board. But let's start out with a broadly accepted proposition—wealthier is healthier—or, even more broadly, individuals with a higher socioeconomic status have better health—and then we'll start going around in circles.

Wealthier People Are Not Necessarily Healthier

We'll start with Ellen Meara, of Harvard Medical School. Her paper is called *Why is Health Related to Socioeconomic Status? The Case of Pregnancy and Low Birth Weight.* She examined pregnancy and health at birth to investigate how socioeconomic status may be related to health. . . .

A limited set of maternal health habits during pregnancy, particularly smoking habits, can explain about half of the correlation between socioeconomic status and low birth weight among white mothers and about one-third of the correlation among black mothers. In contrast, controlling for differential access to medical care and differences in pre-pregnancy maternal health status has no impact on differentials in health outcomes by socioeconomic status.

Well, why do health habits like smoking vary by socioeconomic status factors like education and income? It is most intriguing that Meara finds that education, as measured by differences in knowledge per se, and differences in how pregnant women use common knowledge, account for only about one-third of the difference in health behavior—in this case smoking. The much stronger factor in driving differences in smoking by socioeconomic status appears to be what she terms network effects at the family level, the impact of information and stigma received from those living and working near an individual, in influencing the degree to which those individuals make different investments in both health and education, such as not smoking while pregnant. . . .

Is More Coverage the Right Answer?

Here is the nub of the matter. Insurance coverage can be expanded, though doing so involves dilemmas. Already, a fifth of the uninsured refuse coverage from employers, mainly because it seems too expensive. The costlier private insurance becomes—because, say, government requires coverage of certain treatments—the fewer workers will buy it. Government insurance can fill the void, though this squeezes other programs. But even universal insurance is no panacea, because the real problem is not the uninsured but the poor health of the poor. The two problems aren't the same.

Robert J. Samuelson, *Newsweek*, November 8, 1999.

Meara asks whether Medicaid spending on the poor represents the most effective way to reduce disparities in health. A number of health insurance expansions have lowered adverse outcomes among the poor, such as infant mortality, but through very intensive and very costly medical care interventions at birth, rather than preventing the prevalence of low birth weight and related conditions. She concludes that we may expect too much from prenatal programs for the poor. Infant health disparities by socioeconomic status are largely determined by disparities in health habits, and those disparities exist early in life. Even programs that redistribute income without affecting such third variables as time preferences, self-control and stress may not improve infant health.

Next up, won't national health insurance reduce differences in health outcomes so that, really, money doesn't matter as much? Well, the closest U.S. version of national health insurance and universal coverage is Medicare, for nearly all Americans age 65 and over. But recent work by John Wennberg, Elliott Fisher and Jonathan Skinner, in *Health Affairs*, shows that Medicare spending varies more than twofold among different regions, and those variations persist even after differences in health are corrected for. . . .

What about another international example? Orazio Attanasio, of the University College in London, and Carl Emmerson, of the Institute for Fiscal Studies, studied the relationship between socioeconomic status and health outcomes, or, more particularly, between mortality, health status and wealth. They used data from the British Retirement Survey, controlling for initial health status. Attanasio and Emmerson found that wealth rankings are important determinants of mortality and health outcomes even in a country such as the United Kingdom, with universal government-run health care. . . .

Giving Money to the Poor Does Not Make Them Healthier

However, Jonathan Meer and Harvey Rosen of Princeton, along with Douglas Miller of the University of California at Berkeley, would caution against concluding that dollars count more than doctors and that significant health gains can be made with relatively moderate spending for income transfers to the poor. In their paper, *Exploring the Health-Wealth Nexus*, they use more sophisticated instrumental variables procedures, with inheritance as an instrument for change in wealth. And they find no short-term impact of wealth on health, at least for as long as a five-year period.

If we want to close the health outcomes gap between rich and poor, and simply transferring money directly to poor people won't do the job, why not just throw more subsidies at the health care industry itself, so that more and better health care can be produced and then made available to everyone at lower prices? Well, let's take a look at what Dana Goldman and Darius Lakdawalla of RAND said in that regard.

They started in their paper, *Understanding Health Disparities Against Education Groups*, with the widely accepted consensus view that better educated people are healthier, but then they dug a little deeper to find that health disparities actually increase as the price of health inputs fall. Indeed, government subsidies for health care research, technological progress and, ironically, even universal health insurance, may worsen health inequality over time.

What is really at work here is that the reductions in the price of health care, or expansions in the overall demand for health inputs, disproportionately benefit the well-educated. Technological progress also lowers the quality-adjusted price of health care.

Better Educated People Are Better at Managing Their Own Health

All these price-reducing measures boost the overall level of health investment, which is then reflected in greater disparities across education groups. Those disparities are widest among sicker groups because they consume more health inputs. The chronically ill do learn more by doing, and they gain the most experience in controlling more of their own health investments. But, most of all, more educated people are more productive at managing their own health, and they are the first to adopt and benefit from new patient-intensive technologies.

Goldman and Lakdawalla note that health inputs under an individual's control are more important than medically intensive inputs, and the educated use more self-managed care than the uneducated. So, if we run more escalating rounds of the medical arms race, the less educated will lag further behind and receive smaller shares of—dare I call it— trickle-down health care. But greater levels of schooling do improve health.

An apple a day for the teacher may keep the emergency room doctor away, but do only the dumb die young? Well, Adriana Lleras-Muney of Princeton has a new paper out in

June 2002 called, *The Relationship Between Education and Adult Mortality in the United States.* It suggests not only that more education reduces mortality rates but the effect is much stronger than previously assumed.

For her experiment, she examined States that strengthened their compulsory schooling in child labor laws between 1915 and 1939. Depending on the measure she uses, an additional year of education lowers the probability of dying in the next 10 years by approximately 1.3 to 3.6 percentage points. She concludes that the benefits of education are large enough that we need to consider education policy more seriously as a means to increase health, especially in light of the fact that other factors, such as expenditures on health, have not been proven to be very effective. . . .

Self-Employed People Find Ways to Finance Health Care Without Insurance

Finally, what about the largely unchallenged assumption that greater levels of health insurance coverage must be subsidized for those people who are less likely to be fully insured in order to increase their utilization of health care services and improve their health outcomes. Harvey Rosen and Craig Perry of Princeton, in a paper called *Insurance and the Utilization of Medical Services Among the Self-Employed*, analyzed how the self-employed and wage earners differ with respect to insurance coverage and utilization of various health care services.

They found that even though the self-employed received significantly smaller tax incentives to purchase health insurance and they accordingly are less likely to be insured, the self-employed are able to finance access to care from sources other than insurance. Their relative lack of health insurance does not substantially reduce their utilization of health care services, it does not create economic hardship, or have a negative impact either on their health or the health of their children.

Perry and Rosen suggest that access to health care may be responsible for only a relatively small part of health, with more important determinants being genetics, environment, and human behaviors.

Well, isn't health care, though, at least essential for financial protection against sudden health shocks? Let's turn to

Helen Levy of the University of Chicago, who examined that issue in her April 2000 paper, *The Financial Impact of Health Insurance*. She noted that households may choose to self-insure by accumulating assets instead of buying formal insurance to protect their household consumption levels against health shocks. Levy found that nights spent in the hospital nor new diagnoses of various serious health conditions had a large effect on household consumption. . . .

No Causal Relationship Has Been Established Between Health Insurance and Health

Finally, we turn to Helen Levy again, with colleague David Meltzer of the University of Chicago, who ask, *What Do We Really Know About Whether Health Insurance Affects Health?* in a December 2001 paper. They note that very few of the hundreds of past studies establish a causal relationship between health insurance and health. They are largely dismissive of observational studies that, in their view, do not account for the difficulty of observing truly random variation on health insurance status for causal relationships that run in both directions and for other unobserved factors. . . .

So, after blowing away most of the past studies analyzing health insurance and health, Levy and Meltzer conclude that there may be a small positive effect of health insurance on health outcomes on those populations most likely to be the targets of public coverage expansions, but that there is also evidence that in some cases expansions in health insurance may not result in measurable improvements in health. . . .

Expanding Coverage Is Not the Only Way to Improve the Health of the Uninsured

Levy and Meltzer admit they cannot say which interventions related to health insurance would be most effective in improving health. And they point out that expanding insurance is not the only way to improve health. So it remains unsettled as to whether money aimed at improving health would be better spent on expanded health insurance or other interventions that directly target health or access to medical care, such as inner-city clinics, community-based screening programs, or advertising campaigns to encourage nutrition.

*"What's happening today [2002] is that cost
pressures are being passed around the
system like a hot potato."*

Health Care Spending Is a Serious Problem

Mick L. Diede and Richard Liliedahl

In the following viewpoint, Mick L. Diede and Richard
Liliedahl argue that all the players in the health care system—
providers, consumers, employers, drug and technology companies, insurers, and the government—are responsible for
out-of-control spending. All, therefore, must make sacrifices
to reduce health care costs before it is too late and government intervention is required, they maintain. Diede and
Liliedahl contend that if costs are not controlled, consumers
will see a 55 percent increase in health care costs by the end
of 2006. Mick L. Diede is a principal and actuary in the Atlanta office of Milliman USA, an actuarial consulting firm.
Richard L. Liliedahl is a physician and principal in the firm's
Seattle office.

As you read, consider the following questions:
1. According to the authors, what group will bear the brunt
   of the projected health care increases?
2. Who is the largest purchaser of health care in the
   country, according to Diede and Liliedahl?
3. What do the authors say might happen if lawmakers
   attempt to limit the profits of drug and technology
   companies?

Mick L. Diede and Richard Liliedahl, "Getting on the Right Track," *Managed
Care*, February 2002, pp. 24–33. Copyright © 2002 by MediMedia USA.
Reproduced by permission.

The cost of our health care system is spinning out of control and no one is applying the brakes. While many "solutions" are being offered, they typically address only part of the health care equation, and most often are grounded in a perspective that favors one sector over others. A real solution will, of necessity, involve pain for all players in health care: employers, government, providers, insurers, pharmaceutical and medical technology companies, and consumers.

From our perspective, the best way to regain control is for purchasers and consumers, who have the most to lose in the short term, to join in demanding a resolution that requires the sacrifices that will reduce the rate of increase in health care costs. The alternative—unwanted by most parties—is for the government to step in and mandate its own "solutions."

There is justifiable cause for alarm. Using public data provided by the federal Office of the Actuary, Milliman USA created a model that predicts health care cost increases based on the interdependencies of the key participants in the U.S. health care system. This model integrates the federal data with those collected for Milliman USA's 2001 HMO Intercompany Rate Survey and with more informal surveys of Milliman health care consultants and emerging plan experience to develop assumptions for resource use. Under this model, which also incorporates data from the Milliman USA Health Cost Index, we estimate that per-capita health care costs for all payers—government, insurance carrier, and consumer—will increase 44 percent by 2006, 13 percent higher than what the Office of the Actuary predicts.

By either estimate, the impact will be dramatic and is likely to be felt by consumers first. With premium increases already on the rise, many employers are forcing employees to shoulder more health care costs. As employee premium payments and out-of-pocket spending for noncovered services continue to grow, our models show consumers bearing the brunt of projected increases, with their health care tabs set to increase by 55 percent from 2001 through 2006. This translates into a $2,500 increase in annual household medical spending (premium share and out-of-pocket combined) for a family of four by the end of that period.

Terrorism May Affect Costs

More sobering, these estimates, which assume that current trends continue, may be low and could be adversely affected by a variety of factors. One that has been much discussed but is difficult to pin down is the rise in health care costs associated with acts of terrorism. While there will be increased costs in the short term—especially in some geographic areas—it is unclear how costs five years out will change. Here too, costs are most likely to fall on employers and—eventually—consumers. While insurance companies and HMOs might fail to reach profit objectives in the near term, it's likely they eventually would recover cost increases through higher premiums. Also, job losses increase the number of consumers who must rely on the Consolidated Omnibus Budget Reconciliation Act (COBRA) for health coverage or do without it altogether.

Other forces may come into play. If, for example, more employers begin to adopt strategies such as defined contribution plans, the increase for consumers could be decidedly higher. In a defined contribution scenario, an employer offers employees a set amount of nontaxable benefit dollars to "spend" as they choose. Increasingly, this is a hot topic among employers, and many experts say these plans are gaining in popularity.

When one steps back to look at the entire picture, the first major challenge will be to manage the rate of cost increase, while working to improve quality and access. Keeping costs under control should not mean reduced quality, but this is no easy task.

Reducing the increase in health care spending—or just keeping it at the same level as the growth of the nonhealth care portion of the gross domestic product (GDP)—will require the health care delivery system to spend about 4 percent per year less than projected through 2006, achieving an aggregate saving of 18 percent. This means that all recipients of health care dollars—hospitals, doctors, pharmaceutical and medical equipment companies, long-term care facilities, and home-health providers—will have to find ways to cut back.

Comparing today's situation with that of the early 1990s

underscores the difficulties ahead. In the '90s, everyone thought managed care would reduce health care inflation dramatically, and the early results appeared to validate that assumption. Managed care companies did significantly reduce health care inflation by negotiating lower payment levels to providers and promoting improved quality and efficiency for many health care services. Over time, however, many patients and providers have expressed their disillusionment with managed care's cost-cutting measures, access limitations, and bureaucratic red tape. With market share no longer growing, the pendulum is now swinging back: Many hospitals and physicians are successfully negotiating fee increases well in excess of general inflation to make up for low compensation in recent years. Managed care organizations alone couldn't keep costs down, nor can any other player.

What's happening today [2002] is that cost pressures are being passed around the system like a hot potato. In addition to hospital and physician increases, HMO expenditures on prescription drugs are rising dramatically (more than 18 percent in the past year). The HMOs, in turn, as Milliman's 2001 HMO Intercompany Rate Survey reports, are raising their rates an average of 13 percent to 19 percent, and other insurers are raising rates similarly. Employers, socked with higher premiums, are passing more of the cost along to consumers. The players need to stop the game and figure out a way to play together.

A Fragile Balance

In an ideal world, everyone in the system has a role to play in reducing costs, but in a pragmatic one, not everyone is equally motivated to do so. With consumers, employers, and the government likely to bear the cost increases already in the pipeline, these groups will have the strongest early incentive to push for reductions in health care spending. The operative question is whether they can, together, structure a way to do so.

Keep in mind, however, that they will not be the only constituencies affected by the rise in costs. The U.S. health care system relies on an imperfect balance of stakeholders and their interests. Inflation will affect every party in what is

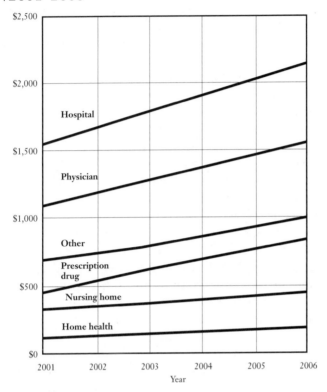

U.S. Per Capita Health Care Expenditures, 2001–2006

Hospital

Physician

Other

Prescription drug

Nursing home

Home health

Year

Milliman USA Estimates

a fragile balance. If the current scenario is allowed to play out unchallenged, everyone stands to lose something:

Employers, who already pay high premiums, will face staggering cost increases. Small employers, many of which already struggle to provide benefits, may be priced out of the market and drop coverage altogether. Those that decide to scale back coverage will lose the competitive recruiting edge that benefits often provide, and risk employee dissatisfaction as well. High health insurance costs also will make it more difficult for U.S. companies to meet shareholder expectations and compete in the global economy.

Consumers, probably, will be the biggest losers. Some will be forced to drop coverage altogether. Those who retain it will bear a substantially larger financial burden and may see their benefits reduced. Either way, consumers will be more likely to forgo care because of its expense, which may result in poorer health and a lower quality of life.

The government, which plays many roles, from regulator to purchaser, will feel the heaviest impact of cost increases when funding coverage for employees and Medicare and Medicaid beneficiaries. As the largest purchaser of health care, the government will shoulder a huge proportion of additional costs, which it will undoubtedly pass on to government employees, taxpayers, and providers of care. At the same time, the government as regulator will come under mounting pressure to take steps to mitigate the rapid cost increases.

Providers, especially institutional facilities, will ultimately experience increased financial pressures, particularly as government reimbursement shrinks. Some, unable to bear the financial burden, will close. Individual providers, whose bargaining power will erode, will be pressured to do more for less.

Managed care organizations and other insurers will be under greater pressure from purchasers to keep costs down. At the same time, they will face demands for higher fees from providers, such as hospitals and physician networks. Some will lose market share as employers self-insure, contract directly with providers, and join purchasing coalitions.

Pharmaceutical and medical technology companies may initially benefit from increased spending but will undoubtedly suffer in the court of public opinion—something we see already—if costs continue to spiral upward and drugs and devices become increasingly unaffordable. Public pressure on lawmakers to create affordable access to drugs and devices will grow, particularly as the population ages. If lawmakers attempt to limit profits, however, drug and technology companies may respond by reducing their investment in research and development. . . .

The irony, despite the practical, economic, and political obstacles to initiating meaningful change, is that all of the system's participants can play several roles in lowering costs without great sacrifice.

The overarching need is for better coordination and more collaboration among participants. One example: Employers need to work with health plans and providers to improve access and quality while controlling costs. Already, we are seeing this happen in some parts of the country, where new types of provider networks are working under quality-driven payment arrangements. Health plans are integral to this type of scheme because they can provide relatively complete data on provider performance and clinical outcomes.

More specifically, one can go sector by sector and find obvious and not-so-obvious practices that can be implemented with relative ease—all of which would dramatically reduce some of the unnecessary expense in health care.

In the consumer sector, for example, the steps are straightforward, much discussed and, at best, ineffectively acted upon. Consumers, sheltered from the true cost of health care by employers who pay the lion's share of the premium and by low copayments, need to become more cost-conscious. In the same vein, they have to be educated to adjust their expectations and to find the right balance between demanding the latest drugs and treatments and first using less-expensive, appropriate tests, procedures, and medications. They also must be taught to recognize the value of healthy lifestyles on a personal level and in terms of lessening demands on the health care system.

Similarly, the employer/purchaser agenda runs along very pragmatic lines. In addition to helping employees understand their role in keeping health care inflation under control, employers should encourage the design of benefit plans that provide incentives to consumers to use health care resources in a responsible and cost-efficient way. Such vehicles include lower copayments for generic drugs, and incentives to use cost-effective, high-quality providers. The importance of carefully planned preventive care in reducing the need for more costly treatments down the road—as well as in improving the quality of life—also needs to be stressed.

Joining forces with other purchasers has proven to be an effective way to bring about change. Coalitions with clout, such as the Midwest Business Group on Health and the Leapfrog Group, have brought about significant change, successfully pushing for higher quality in health care, lower rates, and greater access to services. Also, purchasers must recognize that it is in their interest to support the gathering of statistically meaningful data about quality across employee groups, working with other employers to standardize requests and to limit demands for costly customized data.

The steps that HMOs and other insurers can take parallel, in some respects, the concerns of purchasers—the need for appropriate financial incentives in plan design and for more extensive consumer education aimed at fostering more prudent use of health care services. In addition, insurers have to examine carefully their own practices. It's no secret that administrative complexity increases cost, and carriers should work to streamline routine processes. The Health Insurance Portability and Accountability Act of 1996 promotes standardization of provider-data layouts. Insurers need to capture all the information from a patient encounter, rather than just what is needed to process claims. More complete data sets are the foundation of quality-and-efficiency-improvement studies.

That information, in turn, can be used to create financial incentives for providers, to improve access and quality, and to utilize sensible preventive care and screening tests. Insurers can provide physicians with information about patient compliance with medication and preventive services along with data showing them how they compare to their peers on key quality measures—all of which should serve to improve quality of care.

On the provider side of the equation there are four significant issues to address.

First, providers must accept accountability for resource management. . . . Their task is to advance quality and meet demands of employers and purchasers for improved performance while keeping overall costs under control.

Second, they must accept ownership of quality issues. . . . Physicians and institutional providers must accept these standards or establish their own, and work to improve access and reduce treatment variation through use of evidence-based practice.

Third, providers can work with insurers to improve appropriate drug use by analyzing claims data to identify patients who do not adhere to medication regimens. . . .

Fourth, providers must practice demand and expectation

management. . . . Patients, for instance, bring their doctors articles from the Internet about new treatments or technology they want, or press for an antibiotic when it is not indicated. Physicians need to educate patients about appropriate care and resist the temptation to give in to pressure.

Reining in the spiraling cost of drugs and new technology, two significant contributors to health care inflation, will not be easy. Milliman's 2001 HMO Intercompany Rate Survey shows spending on pharmaceuticals alone accounted for 26 percent of HMO medical cost increases over the last year. . . .

Far and away, the most contentious element in the health care equation is the role to be played by government. Controversial practices, such as coverage mandates for expensive treatments, will often increase cost without improving quality of care. As a purchaser and the overseer of Medicare and other programs, the government should design benefit plans that encourage consumers to use resources wisely and develop reimbursement approaches for hospitals and other providers that include incentives to treat patients in the least expensive, most appropriate setting.

Laws designed to protect patients or expand their choices often cost them money, and the right balance must be found between these priorities. At this writing, Congress and the president are debating the merits of patient-rights legislation, which will give enrollees more legal recourse if care is denied, but would, according to Congressional Budget Office estimates, raise premiums about 4 percent. [As of September 2002, no Patients' Rights Bill had been approved.]

With pressure for cost containment building and the price of inaction high, the imperative to act is strong. Delay will create pressure for government action—something sure to divide the diverse interests within health care. The struggle for favorable regulatory position—and survival—under a government-mandated solution will not be pretty.

The complexity of our health care landscape and of the relationships among its players does not support simple solutions. As in the past, the debate about controlling health care costs will undoubtedly incline toward blame, when what's really important is recognizing the critical role of interdependence in this delicate balancing act.

> *"It is true that health care will consume a quarter . . . of national resources within a generation or so, but we can well afford that—and without giving up anything else."*

Health Care Spending Is Not a Serious Problem

Charles R. Morris

In the following viewpoint, Charles R. Morris argues that the conventional picture of American health care is completely wrong. Health care is not a drain on the economy; it is a highly productive industry that pays good wages and is needed by everyone, he claims. Health care spending and the economic growth it provides will continue to increase for the next twenty-five years or so, he maintains, because it is driven by baby boomers just entering their health care consuming years. Charles R. Morris is a financial expert and author of opinion pieces appearing in the *New York Times*, the *Wall Street Journal*, and *Atlantic Monthly*.

As you read, consider the following questions:
1. According to Morris, why is America's health care bill larger than other countries'?
2. How much did health care workers make in 1950?
3. Where will money for increased health care spending come from, according to the author?

Charles R. Morris, "Health Spending Is Soaring. What's So Bad About That?" *Medical Economics*, vol. 77, March 6, 2000. Copyright © 2000 by Thompson Medical Economics. Reproduced by permission.

The conventional wisdom is that runaway health care costs are a major threat to the US economy. Government statistics show that they have been rising faster, usually much faster, than the overall rate of inflation for almost as long as we've kept track of such things. The spread of HMOs and other kinds of managed care slowed the pace of growth for a few years in the mid-1990s, but collapsing profit margins have forced almost all insurers to file for big premium increases. Within the next 25 years or so, according to most recent estimates, health care could account for as much as 25 percent of the nation's spending.

Sharply rising costs are a telltale sign of low productivity, which is why analysts are so worried about health care: It looks like an abysmally unproductive sector eating up resources that could otherwise be devoted to increasing national wealth. The industry is an awkward public-private amalgam, with about half of all spending cycled through government accounts. Stories of waste and inefficiency are rampant, and Canada, England, and Germany get by with only half to three-quarters as much spending on health care.

Not only conservative entitlement scourges are worried. To policy wonks health care "reform" is shorthand for cutting costs. When President Bill Clinton introduced his ill-fated health care reform program, in 1993, he said that curbing spending—without, naturally, hurting quality—was essential for "our competitiveness, our whole economy, the integrity of the way our government works, and, ultimately, our living standards."

But there is another side to the story. This viewpoint will argue that the conventional picture of American health care is almost completely wrong, even taking into account the turbulence that currently afflicts the industry. In reality health care, or a very large sector of it, is a high-productivity, high-technology industry that is a good employer and pays above-average wages. America's health care bill is larger than other countries' bills, but we buy more health care, and spending trends in almost all the other developed countries are much the same as in ours, although with a time lag. It is true that health care will consume a quarter, or even more, of national resources within a generation or so, but we can well afford that—and without giving up anything else.

Although the data are very sketchy, most health care costs have quite possibly been going down for a long time. It is health-care spending that is rising, which is quite a different thing. As the personal-computer industry demonstrates, falling costs and improved performance usually induce more spending, not less. In the same way, by any reasonable standard of measurement—prices, outcomes, side effects, recovery time—the cost-effectiveness of cartilage surgery, cardiac bypasses, angioplasty, hip and knee replacements, noninvasive diagnostics, whole new generations of pharmaceuticals, and even mental health interventions has improved dramatically. Cataract surgery used to be a dangerous operation, requiring as long as a week in the hospital for only marginal improvements in vision. Now it's a virtually painless hour-long outpatient procedure that usually restores near-normal sight; not surprisingly, the pool of potential customers is vastly larger. In any other industry that would be hailed as a triumph; in health care it sets off alarm bells.

Modern Medicine Is Affordable

The primary accusation against modern medicine is not that it doesn't work but that it's an unproductive drain on the economy. If we "were able through health reform to achieve a level of spending comparable to other countries," according to a Commerce Department report of several years ago, "the United States could save about 4 percent of GDP. Those savings could be reallocated to investments in other areas . . . thus enhancing the US competitive position."

Sherry Glied, a young economist at Columbia University, argues that this conventional view is mostly nonsense. "What do they want us to spend it on?" she asks. Certainly, it's hard to argue that America is an underconsuming nation. This is a country in which new houses are half again as big as they were 20 years ago, and bursting with gadgets; where citizens drag their sagging bellies from VCRs to $30,000 four-wheel-drive sport-utility vehicles; and where a book like Juliet Schor's *The Overspent American: Why We Want What We Don't Need* is a best-seller. There are plenty of poor people in America, but that is mostly a problem of distribution, not of resources. A scandalously high number of Americans are without health insurance because of a lack of political will, not of economic capacity.

Worries over a shift of resources from the "productive" economy into health care also ignore the world-beating competitiveness of America's pharmaceutical and medical-equipment sectors. For instance, the profile of Medtronic, a leading manufacturer of medical devices, looks very much like Intel's 10 years ago. Medtronic's sales are about the same as Intel's were then and are rising about as fast, and the company spends about the same percentage of revenues on research and development. . . . About 40 percent of Medtronic's sales are to overseas markets, which is about average in the medical-equipment industry.

In any case, the "squeezing out" argument is grossly overstated. Glied points out that the share of national income devoted to food and health care combined hasn't changed for 50 years. But we spend a lot less than we used to on food and a lot more on health care—just as we spend a lot less on clothing and a lot more on housing. Meanwhile, overall income growth has freed up mega-resources for Arnold Schwarzenegger movies, stealth bombers, and interactive pornography. Careful projections by government researchers in 1992 showed that absent "reform," the twin forces of technology and demographics would drive health care spending to about 27 percent of GDP by 2020, and to about 32 percent by 2030. The projections assumed a very modest economic growth rate of 1.1 percent a year through 2030—a much lower rate than we actually achieved in the 1990s. Remarkably, though, even under this assumption of slow growth, the projections show the nonhealth care sectors of the economy continuing to grow, at a rate of 0.8 percent a year. In other words, since health care is still a relatively minor fraction of the economy, it can grow very fast for a long time and yet leave plenty of income for even more VCRs and behemoth cars.

Glied also challenges the notion that health care is unusually inefficient. "Relative to what?" she asks. "Universities are pretty inefficient, and so are banks. Everyone complains about health care overhead, but it's about the same as in most other industries, maybe even lower. There is this notion that health care should be only doctors and nurses, but nobody thinks that General Motors is just the guys on the production line.". . . Although there's plenty of waste and fraud, Glied says, it's not a large percentage of the total, and the cost of rooting it out might be almost as great as the savings.

Another favorite nostrum, reducing medical spending in the last year of a person's life, is probably a blind alley as well. Michael Lesch, a cardiologist at St. Luke's-Roosevelt Hospital, says, "If I knew which patients were in their last year of life, maybe I would treat them differently." Bruce Vladeck, who ran the Medicare program during much of the Clinton Administration, says that 27 percent of Medicare dollars are spent on people in their last year of life, but only a small fraction of that amount is spent on people whom medical professionals expect to die. In fact, recent data suggest that people with slow-acting terminal cancers or degenerative heart disease are now much more likely than they once would have been to die in hospices or at home, but such palliative care is also surprisingly expensive, especially if it involves round-the-clock nursing. Vladeck says, "We should do a much better job than we do in managing end-of-life treatment, but it won't be a big money-saver."

The Myth That Health Care Is "Nonproductive"

To a great extent the bad reputation of health care stems from economic scoring systems that track what's easiest to count. Gouging coal out of mountains to run power plants so that we can waft cool air over the brows of investment bankers is totted up as "industrial production"—an unambiguous increase in national wealth, like Jet Skis and video games. But new hips that allow people to walk, intraocular implants that restore their vision, coronary artery stents that put them back to work, are classified as nonproductive "services" that somehow make us poorer. . . .

At the end of the day the problem with health care spending is not that it's inefficient but that it's redistributive. Each year the small fraction of people who are very sick account for the lion's share of health care spending. They are different people, of course, from year to year, and the odds are that all of us, once or twice in our lives, will take our turns as mega-medical consumers. Since none but the very wealthiest families can sustain the cost of big-ticket medical episodes, the risk has to be partially socialized, either privately through insurance or publicly through the tax system. I may not want to help pay for your heart attack, but I'll need you to kick in, one way or another, for the cost of my cancer.

Whatever minimally adequate health care financing system we eventually muddle toward will inevitably contain leveling components. Families on the lower third or so of the economic ladder simply can't afford the full cost of adequate private medical insurance, and neither can most marginal employers. Americans don't like statist solutions, usually with good reason, so we will maintain our commitment to the current mixed public-private framework, with all its ideological messiness. But even if most providers are private companies, the public sector will inevitably play a larger role in paying for an ever-expanding range of "basic" health care services.

Politicians don't like facing up to issues like these—better to pretend that the financing issues will disappear if we just crack down on waste and fraud. But it's wrong to assume that tax-financed health care is inherently less productive or socially beneficial than private-sector spending—indeed, in our Jerry Springer, consumer-binge culture, the opposite may well be true. Moreover, a growing health care sector may carry positive benefits for the American job market.

The Health Care Career Machine

A decade ago Robert Reich, the Secretary of Labor in the first Clinton Administration, sounded the alarm over a bifurcating American job market, foreseeing a spreading income gap between knowledge workers with one or more degrees from top universities and the great mass of workers stuck in dead-end jobs. Health care is a refreshing exception to Reich's paradigm. St. Luke's-Roosevelt operates a huge outpatient surgery center on New York's West Side that—to a visitor with expectations tuned by *The Hospital* and similar movies—seems impressively efficient. Service is brisk, queues are short, and a scoreboardlike electronic screen allows friends and relatives to track patients' progress through prep, surgery, and recovery. The majority of the workers I saw were young people of color, handling millions of dollars' worth of high-tech equipment with competence and professionalism. . . .

The Health Cost Containment Crisis Is Overstated

The casual newspaper reader . . . could be forgiven for assuming that medical care cost containment is one of the most urgent tasks facing the nation. The belief in the importance of this task seems to rest on a few facts: (1) The level of spending on health care in the United States greatly exceeds that of any other country. At the same time, U.S. mortality rates do not compare favorably with those of other countries, suggesting that the United States does not buy anything useful with its extra spending on health care. Some people believe that administrative waste is a prime source of the extra spending. Others believe that even if the United States is getting value for its health care dollar, high health expenditures damage the American competitive position. (2) The growth rate of health spending exceeds the growth rate in the economy, resulting in an ever-larger share of gross domestic product (GDP) devoted to health care and, consequently, a smaller share of the pie available for other worthy activities. . . .

I argue that the rhetoric about the urgency for cost containment may well be overstated. . . .

Why is growth in medical care spending cause for concern? After all, many sectors of the economy have grown over the years; the computer and telecommunications industries are two obvious examples. Indeed, just as we spend more on health care than any other country, we may well spend more per person on personal computers, fax machines, and cellular telephones as well. Yet no one I know is calling for cost containment for these industries.

Joseph F. Newhouse, *Health Affairs*, October 29, 2001.

Health care was once a low-wage, dead-end field, with doctors roosting comfortably at the top of a job pyramid filled out with underpaid nurses, orderlies, and aides. In 1950 health care workers earned about two-thirds of the average wage. By the mid-1990s, however, with rising capital investment per worker, health care wages had risen to about 109 percent of the economy-wide average. In addition, US pharmaceutical and medical-equipment companies, with annual sales of about $170 billion, pay better than the average manufacturer, because of medicine's demanding quality requirements. Health care spending, moreover, unlike spending for cars, television sets, clothing, and oil, tends to stay home. The alarm over rising health care spending suggests that the money is somehow dribbling away into outer space rather than being recycled into the pockets of a growing new class of professional workers.

These are turbulent times for health care. Price pressures have left doctors feeling rushed, harried, and second-guessed. Tens of thousands of articles are published in medical journals each year. Drug companies flog their products in "Ask your doctor" television ads. Boomers surf the Web for the latest treatments for their aging moms. Medical practices jostle with fast food chains for space in Florida's strip malls. Even as they orchestrate round after round of Medicare cutbacks, both political parties are moving toward adding a very expensive pharmaceutical benefit to the basic Medicare package.

A Time of Turbulence and Transition

Health care is undergoing a fundamental transition. The old pattern of solo-practitioner medicine has been irrevocably destroyed by the burgeoning of medical technology, but a workable new model has yet to emerge. Cardiologist Michael Lesch asks, "How do you keep the benefits of the marketplace—innovation, competition, lower prices, patient choice—without its drawbacks? Do you think Ford cares whether you really need three cars? And do you think drug companies really care whether you need the medicine? They just want you to buy it. How do we stay a profession with some market elements, and not become a business that's just out for profits?"

One response has been the evidence-based medicine movement. Scott Weingarten, MD, is the president of Zynx, a research and consulting firm that specializes in establishing evidence-based health care management practices. "There are things that science shows work, and work well," Weingarten says. "But there are big gaps between what we actually do and what we ought to be doing—and that includes treatment in the finest academic medical centers in the land. Technologies that don't work, or are actually harmful, are being used throughout the United States.". . .

The case for evidence-based medicine seems irrefutable, though it is too often promoted just as a way to cut spending. But there is no intrinsic reason why good medicine should cost less: For every improper practice eliminated, there may well be another useful intervention from which patients will benefit. . . .

Delivering high-quality, science-based medicine to an aging population will grow ever more complex. Patients with multiple chronic disorders won't match the "pure" cases selected for clinical trials, and the growing list of plausible pharmaceutical interventions greatly increases the risk of dangerous drug interactions. Effective management of an older, sicker population will require vast new investments in information technology just to begin. . . .

In short, although the vague outlines of the evidence-based and information-linked health care system of the future may be taking shape, there are huge gaps, and no obvious ways to bridge them. The only certainty is that the ride will be bumpy—and very expensive.

Increased Spending Is Inevitable

Almost half a century ago the oldest baby boomers entered first grade; from 1950 through 1970 the school-age population (5 to 19) nearly doubled, and school spending after inflation quadrupled. And those boomers didn't vote.

Ever since the end of World War II the national economy has been defined by the life passages of the baby boomers. Only compare the smooth seas of the '90s—when boomers settled into placid, productive middle age—with the turmoil of the 1970s, when unskilled boomers poured into the job market. Yet policy wonks still treasure the delusion that we as a nation will somehow decide what share of resources should be claimed by health care, when the demographic facts have already decided it for us.

Good planning may help around the edges, but the shift to a health care–based economy will inevitably be a messy one, complicated by the inevitable shift of resources toward the public and nonprofit sectors. One consolation is that almost all our international competitors will be undergoing the same kinds of demographic upheaval, often more severe than ours.

Where will the health care dollars come from? Some will come from the boomers' own pockets. Expect a more sharply tiered medical system, with basic coverage for all seniors and elite care for those who can afford it. Boomers will find the money by retiring later, working harder, liquidating assets, and borrowing against their houses. Much of the money will come from steeper payroll taxes (and a lot of the people paying them will be working in health care, or selling things to people who do). And some of it will come from holding down fees paid to doctors and hospitals. The medical establishment got a huge windfall when Medicare was first passed, and part of that will be clawed back in the decades ahead. It's too bad that different doctors got the windfall, but there's nothing in the Constitution about generational equity. Paying off the national debt would help a lot, too. Then the government could start borrowing again when boomer medical spending peaks, spreading the costs over a couple of generations.

A leading medical analyst recently wrote that "doubling or tripling health care expenditures would be intolerable." But in fact the doubling or tripling of health care spending is a virtual certainty. As Gen-Xers would say, "Get over it!" Let's start thinking about how to make the transition no more traumatic than it has to be.

Periodical Bibliography

The following articles have been selected to supplement the diverse views presented in this chapter.

Drew E. Altman and Larry Levitt — "The Sad History of Health Care Cost Containment as Told in One Chart," *Health Affairs*, January 23, 2002.

Julie Appleby — "Finger Pointers Can't Settle On Who's to Blame for Health Casts," *USA Today*, August 2, 2002.

Business Week — "How to Cover America's Uninsured," August 14, 2000.

Tommy Denton — "Health Care: Not Just a Market Commodity," *Fort Worth Star-Telegram*, January 6, 1998.

Ronald W. Dworkin — "The Cultural Revolution in Health Care," *Public Interest*, Spring 2000.

Eli Ginzberg and Panos Minogiannis — "Providing Universal Coverage Under National Health Insurance," *Western Journal of Medicine*, April 2000.

Howard Gleckman — "Health Care Choice at a Price," *Business Week*, May 6, 2002.

Devon M. Herrick — "Five Myths About the Uninsured in America," *National Center for Policy Analysis Brief*, September 20, 2000.

Michael McCarthy — "Fragmented US Health Care System Needs Major Reform," *Lancet*, March 10, 2001.

Joel E. Miller — "A Perfect Storm: The Confluence of Forces Affecting Health Care Coverage," National Coalition on Health Care, November 2001.

John Moser — "The Golden Age of Health Care," John M. Ashbrook Center for Public Affairs, July 2001.

Linda O. Prager — "The World's Best Health Care Can Be Pretty Mediocre," *American Medical News*, May 17, 1999.

Richard Service — "Reform and Reality," *Business & Health*, November 1998.

Barbara Starfield — "Is U.S. Health Care Really the Best in the World?" *Journal of the American Medical Association*, July 26, 2000.

CHAPTER 2

How Has Managed Care Affected the Health Care System?

Chapter Preface

In the 1970s the United States was rapidly sliding into a recession, and medical spending was growing faster than the economy. Medicare (which provides basic health care for the elderly and disabled) and Medicaid (which provides health care for low-income individuals) were both signed into law in 1965 and proved to be expensive. The medical insurance available to most Americans not covered by either government program was a traditional plan that typically paid whatever their doctor or hospital charged. No one—not the patient, the doctor, or the hospitals—had any incentive to control costs. However, in 1970, Minnesota neurologist Paul Ellwood and Stanford University management professor Alain C. Enthoven developed the health maintenance organization (HMO) concept that promised to curb the rise in health care spending and shift significant future spending from the government to the private sector.

The original HMO plan that Ellwood and Enthoven described to then-president Richard M. Nixon consisted of physician-driven organizations that would provide patients with comprehensive, coordinated medical care for a prearranged, prepaid monthly fee. The organizations would compete based on price and quality of care. Data on patient outcomes would be made public on a regular basis so that patients could determine which HMOs were performing best. Ellwood and Enthoven maintained that their competitive HMO plan would promote high quality medical care and accountability and bring soaring health care inflation under control.

Thus, managed care became part of the U.S. health care system in 1973, when President Nixon signed into law the Health Maintenance Organization Assistance Act. The Nixon administration's faith in managed care was so strong that the act included offers of government grants to help new HMOs get started. Managed care got off to a slow start, however, and few grants were awarded in 1973. Contrary to Ellwood's and Enthoven's initial predictions, by the end of the 1970s, only about 5 percent of Americans were enrolled in managed care arrangements. However, enrollment increased from 9 million in 1980 to 36 million in 1990. By 1996, nearly 74 percent of eligible Americans were members of a prepaid, managed care health plan. Soon it became obvious that managed care was a significant factor in controlling costs, just as Ellwood and Enthoven had anticipated. "The first phase has shifted power from physicians and insurers to large-group purchasers of medical services [HMOs]. This has reduced the growth of expenditures by about $500 billion."

Unfortunately, as managed care in the United States grew, it changed significantly from the concept that Ellwood and Enthoven had laid out for President Nixon. The 1990s brought on an era of mergers and acquisitions that created health care giants and giant problems along with them. In 1990, Cigna Corporation acquired Equicor, a joint venture of the Equitable Life Assurance Society of the U.S. and Hospital Corporation of America. Travelers Corporation and Metropolitan Life Insurance Company merged their respective health insurance operations to form MetraHealth Companies, Inc., soon after. Then UnitedHealthCare Corporation bought MetraHealth. "There's a huge irony in the whole thing," Enthoven said. "By HMO, we meant medical groups or physician-created independent practice organizations. But when people say HMO today, they think Aetna, Cigna, UnitedHealthCare. They're all insurance companies." According to Ellwood, that is the crux of the HMO problem. "Unfortunately, the [large-group] purchasers [of medical services] neglected the other component of the HMO proposal, that is, quality and competition." He added, "For those of us who devoted ourselves to reshaping the health system—and where our motives were typical of many physicians, trying to make the health system better for patients—the thing has been a profound disappointment." But he remains hopeful: "The next phase of the evolution will involve another power shift. This time consumers and patients will gain the upper hand by exercising choices based on objective comparisons of quality."

The authors in the following chapter debate some of the issues that make managed care controversial. They explore the challenges that managed care, born of recession and inflationary health care costs in the 1970s, will face in the twenty-first century.

"Clearly, the managed care system, as it is currently constructed, creates ethical conflicts of such magnitude that conscientious physicians feel forced to compromise their personal integrity to survive."

Managed Care Has Harmed the Health Care System

Edmund D. Pellegrino

Edmund D. Pellegrino asserts in the following viewpoint that managed care is ethically suspect. He argues that managed care has harmed the health care system by forcing physicians to choose between their patients and their employer—the HMO. Pellegrino further maintains that under managed care, physicians can no longer advocate against the system on behalf of their patients because the physicians themselves have become part of the system. Edmund D. Pellegrino is emeritus professor of medicine and medical ethics at Georgetown University and a senior research scholar at the Kennedy Institute of Ethics.

As you read, consider the following questions:

1. According to Pellegrino, upon what does the moral status of any system of managed care depend?
2. Pellegrino says that conflicts of loyalty are built into the managed care system in order to achieve what end?
3. In the author's opinion, why is managed care biased against technology?

Edmund D. Pellegrino, "Managed Care at the Bedside: How Do We Look in the Moral Mirror?" *Kennedy Institute of Ethics Journal*, vol. 7, December 1997, pp. 321–30. Copyright © 1997 by The Johns Hopkins University Press. Reproduced by permission.

The ethical issues in managed care can be examined at three levels—at the bedside, which centers chiefly on the patient-physician relationship; at the managerial or corporate level, which centers on the relationships of managers, corporate boards and officers, and investors to patients; and at the social level, which centers on the way a society responds to the ill, disabled, and vulnerable in its midst. Managed care as it is operated today poses serious ethical questions at all three levels.

This essay confines itself to the ethical issues at the bedside—i.e., on the way this particular form of health care organization affects the sick and those who profess to help them. . . .

These "bedside" issues cannot be fully separated from the ethical issues at the managerial and societal levels. If harm results, the moral complicity of corporate officers and investors, as well as society as a whole, cannot be escaped. Those who manage, invest in, and profit from managed care cannot escape moral complicity for harms that occur at the bedside.

Generically, managed care is morally neutral. It refers simply to any system of health care that aims at constraints on the clinician's management of care to achieve some stated purpose. That purpose may take many forms—the quality of care provided to an individual patient, the personal well-being of the patient, the containment of costs, the welfare of society, or the making of profit. Some of these objectives are morally sound; some are morally reprehensible. Ultimately, the moral status of any system of managed care will depend upon the purpose, the means employed to attain that purpose, and the priorities between and among purposes or means when they conflict with each other.

In all of these variations of managed care, and in actual practice, one ordering principle provides the moral *sine qua non*; it is the primacy of the moral obligation of health care professions to act in the best interests of the person who is ill. This is the moral principle of beneficence contained in traditional codifications of the physician's obligations. This is, has always been, and must remain the telos of the healing relationship, the end built into the nature of medicine and without which it becomes something other than a healing relationship.

The moral test, therefore, of a managed care system is not in the balance sheet of the HMO nor in the dividend reports of the investor nor in the bonus to the "provider" nor even in the costs saved, bed days reduced, efficiency gained, or productivity improved. The moral test of any system of care is its impact on the patient for whom the system is presumably designed and on the physician from whom the patient seeks help.

First of all, none of what follows is a denial of the reality of economics as a constraining force on medicine. The real issue is how to relate the fact of economics to the demands of ethics. Throughout, I shall maintain that when they are in conflict, ethics takes precedence over economics, but cannot ignore it. . . .

Thus, an economically sensitive physician, faced with two treatments of equal effectiveness and benefit for her patient, should choose the one that is less costly. This is a moral obligation since the physician acts unjustly if he knowingly wastes the patient's money. In addition, physicians have responsibilities to use not only a patient's resources efficiently, but society's as well. Even when resources are limited, there are morally sound and morally unsound ways of confronting the dilemmas of clinical choice. Under certain conditions rationing can be morally justified so long as these conditions are set by ethics and not economics. . . .

Physicians are under moral obligation not to offer or provide treatments that are unnecessary, especially when treatment is futile. This is not simply for economic reasons. Unnecessary treatment is morally wrong because it violates the obligatory canons of good medicine, imposes costs without reason, and exposes patients to risks without proportional benefits. If physicians in the past had more assiduously observed the moral duty to avoid unneeded treatment, much of the impetus to managed care would not have existed. . . .

In the past, and at present, care has been "managed," albeit indirectly, by measures aimed at enhancing quality—e.g. tissue committees, postmortem examinations, pharmacy and therapeutics committees, drug formularies, morbidity and mortality conferences, patient care committees, and the hospital and residency accreditation processes. These and like measures illustrate that managed care can be used for purposes other than cost containment. It shows too that physicians can accept managing care if the patient's welfare is the primary goal, even if such management limits their discretionary latitude in clinical decisions. To be sure, these measures can be expanded and improved upon. It is politically and morally offensive for physicians to resist managing care if it is designed for the patient's good. Anyone familiar with the dark side of unfettered clinical decision making will recognize the value of patient- and quality-oriented managed care. Unfortunately, this is not the driving force of managed care as it operates today in the United States.

The Dilemma of Divided Loyalty

In any managed care system, the most fundamental and ubiquitous moral dilemma at the bedside is the dilemma of divided loyalty—i.e., pitting the welfare of the patient against the welfare of the organization, the physician, or the other plan subscribers. The physician who works in a managed care organization is financially and factually an employee. She accepts remuneration presumably to serve the needs of the employer. This is a contractual relationship, and it carries responsibilities to the employer and to the investors who make the employer's business possible by risking their capital. This contractual obligation conflicts with a morally determined patient-physician relationship, which gives primacy to the well-being of the patient.

In its strong form, the ideology of managed care asserts that the person-oriented ethics of traditional medical ethics must give way to population ethics, to a concern for the impact of every clinical decision on the availability of resources to others covered by the same system. On this view, the physician become *primarily* an advocate for society rather than for his patient. This is the model of implicit rationing in which the physician as gatekeeper decides who is to receive scarce resources, with or without socially imposed criteria for choice. "Social ethics" takes the place of the traditional ethic of individual patient care.

A weaker form of this model requires at least equal concern for the good of the population as for the good of the individual patient. Here the physician is expected to balance the moral claims of her own patient against those of other plan participants and societal need in general. This model also depends upon implicit rationing in which the final decisions on allocation at the bedside belong to physicians. In both versions, strong and weak, the patient is at the mercy of the physician's assessment of her relative worth in the competition for limited research.

Physicians Are Sometimes Forced to Lie

Although lately challenged, managed care organizations have sought to further the interests of profit or the population at large by imposing "gag" rules of various degrees of stringency on physician employees. While legislation has been developing to limit specific "gag" clauses, there is still the subtler problem of not telling the whole truth. By this I mean that managed care gatekeepers may not feel obliged or expected to tell a patient that the treatment his plan will pay for, or the surgeon, hospital, or laboratory it contracts with, are not the preferred ones for *this* patient's illness. The patient's freedom of choice and autonomy are thus violated without his knowing it. The physician fails to fulfill his fiduciary obligations to be honest and to enhance patient autonomy. Simultaneously, he silently sanctions a lesser standard of care than he would if he were free to make the decisions he thought best for his patient.

In addition, to serve his patient best, some physicians are tempted to lie—i.e., to ratchet up the severity of an illness or to place it in a diagnostic category more favorably received by the managed care plan of the pre-admission auditor. How far may the truth be shaded, or stretched, in the interest of an individual patient? Some would say not at all. Others might hold that the restrictions are unjust in the first place and therefore there is no moral obligation to respect them. Others would argue that we must not deceive others even to serve the good of a patient. However stringently or loosely one regards the obligation of truth telling, any system of care that makes truth telling an obstacle to beneficence is suspect on the face of it.

Some have suggested that these conflicts of loyalty can, for the most part, be avoided if physicians themselves become insurers, or "fund-holders". Theoretically, on this view, it is presumed that doctors who have more control over allocation decisions for individual patients, or local communities of patients, will act more beneficently than managers or bureaucrats. Without disparaging the characters or intentions of physicians, the presumption is a precarious one indeed. If physicians share the risks of fiscal loss, this fact will consciously or unconsciously shape their decisions. When the plans involve profit as well, the danger of loss is accentuated in direct proportion to magnitude of gains or losses.

Moreover, when physicians are stakeholders, they become part of the managed care plan—i.e., of a corporate entity. The patient loses his advocate with the system since the physician is unlikely to advocate the patient's case against his own interests. At least, when the physician is an employee rather than an owner of an interest, he can make common cause with the patient against the system. Confident assurances that patients can be protected against injustices by grievance mechanisms are so unrealistic as to verge on the ridiculous. Patients in need of care, patients dissatisfied with decisions being made, or those being denied needed care are hardly in a position to initiate, much less to pursue, a grievance process. Such a process might be of some use retrospectively to patients seeking retribution for harm done, but it is an unrealistic safeguard at the time the injustice is being perpetrated.

Young Physicians Know Only Managed Care

Clearly, the managed care system, as it is currently constructed, creates ethical conflicts of such magnitude that conscientious physicians feel forced to compromise their personal integrity to survive. Failure to "accommodate" holds the threat of being stricken from the list of "providers" or penalized financially. When the penetrance of managed care is in the range of 40–50 percent of the insured, the threat to survival is not imaginary. The result often is that the more sensitive and humane physicians choose to retire or to move out of direct patient care. This is self-defeating since it leaves the field to those who are willing to compromise.

To this we must add the fact that the youngest physicians are being socialized and professionalized into the managed care ideology. Not having experienced other forms of medicine, it is difficult for them to see why there are objections. They believe the evils of the indemnity and fee-for-service systems of the past were even greater. The issue is not choosing the better of two bad alternatives, but designing a system that is morally defensible by the standard of its impact on the care of sick persons—presumably those who should be the beneficiaries of the system.

It must be clear that the conflicts of loyalty outlined above are built into managed care to achieve its end of cost containment. They may or may not contain costs. There are also non-dollar costs that significantly affect the quality and satisfaction of the "care" provided by managed care plans. . . .

Non-Dollar Costs: The Care of the Patient

One serious non-dollar cost is the chaotic nature of patient-physician relationships in managed care settings. Discontinuity is more the rule than continuity. The physician one encounters is a matter of random meetings conditioned by physicians' work schedules rather than patient need. The clear assumption is that one physician is as good as any other. The personal "chemistry" of the therapeutic relationship is given short shrift. Over an eight-hour shift, patients may have to report their stories to a succession of nurses and physicians "on call," none of whom seems to have communicated with the other.

The dangers of discontinuity go beyond mere inconvenience. They constitute real dangers to the patient. Vital information may be missing, misinformation and negative attitudes may be transmitted in what passes for "communication" between one physician "passing the torch" to another. Doctors are now shift workers, increasingly less committed to the patient and more to the schedule of both shift and productivity. Fewer physicians see patients as their personal responsibility but rather as the responsibility of the organization.

Moreover, the "productivity" schedules imposed on outpatient visits do not foster confidence nor permit getting to the root of a problem unless it is obvious in the first few minutes. It is difficult indeed to establish an effective patient-physician relationship in 15-minute, random, and intermittent office visits. . . .

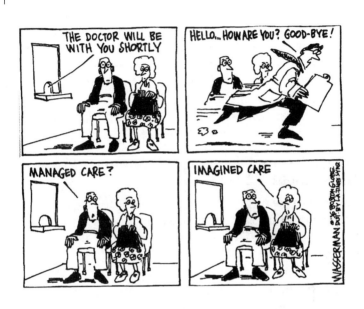

Wasserman. © 1996 by Tribune Media Services. Reprinted with permission.

Another non-dollar cost is the conversion of generalists into marginal specialists and specialists into marginal generalists. To save the costs of referrals, physicians should do more themselves. The generalist is invited to do a little orthopedics here, a dash of office gynecology there, and a soupçon of neurology. Time, after all, will tell whether a specialist is needed. The specialist, on the other hand, can treat a minor respiratory infection, migraine headache, or diarrhea for a while. If it does not go away, then she can refer the patient to a generalist, who starts all over again. All of this adds up to the creep of incompetence. Marginalizing the expertise of either specialist or generalist is a dangerous legitimation of clinical presumptuousness, the costs of which are yet to be measured in missed or delayed diagnoses and increases in disability, suffering, and patient frustration.

To be sure, some of these hassles and harassments were present with indemnification systems and fee-for-service practice. But in the past, such difficulties were recognized as lapses in good care. The finger of guilt could be pointed directly and legitimately at the physician who had personal responsibility for what happened to the patient. Managed care systems, however, legitimate these harassments. They are justified as necessary "inconveniences" legitimized by presumed dollar savings. This, we are told, is necessary to forestall the national economic disaster of spending too much on health care. We do not seem equally worried about our more egregious overspending on self-indulgence, recreation, costs of sports, entertainment, and the like.

Managed Care Discourages Innovative Technology

Even more disturbing among the non-dollar costs is the marginalization and gradual disenfranchisement of segments of the population—the aged, the chronically ill, the underinsured. . . .

The same kind of danger lies in the bias of managed care against medical technology. This verges on a new Luddite movement in which research in currently nontreatable diseases is implicitly discouraged since it will only prolong lives in people who must ultimately die anyway. Measured in terms of increased longevity and improved quality of life, however, effective technologies may well be "worthwhile." What we as a society consider "worthwhile" reflects on the kind of society we want to be. All technology must not be lumped together, therefore, under the heading of "unnecessary care at the end of life.". . .

Managed care is not per se evil. It can be a morally creditable enterprise, but if, and only if, it is designed to serve the needs of those among us who are ill—or will be ill—and that is all of us. As it exists today, it does not meet this moral criterion.

"Almost every U.S. health trend has been positive during the decade of managed care. And, after rising . . . for most of the 1980s, the cost of health care has stabilized."

Managed Care Has Helped the Health Care System

Gregg Easterbrook

In the following viewpoint, Gregg Easterbrook contends that managed care has helped the health care system by keeping Americans healthier while it successfully controls costs. Americans are living longer thanks to managed care's emphasis on preventative medicine, he maintains. In addition, the feared rationing of expensive but proven procedures like bypass surgery and organ transplants has never materialized. Easterbrook insists that pressure from HMOs was responsible for a substantial drop in physician and hospital fees from 1993 to 2000, making health care more affordable and accessible to more people. Gregg Easterbrook is a writer for *The New Republic*.

As you read, consider the following questions:

1. According to the author, why must the majority of physicians and hospitals accept managed care?
2. In Easterbrook's opinion, what was the reason for the establishment of HMOs?
3. Why are denied claims less of a problem now than in the past, according to Easterbrook?

Gregg Easterbrook, "How to Love Your HMO: Managing Fine," *The New Republic*, March 20, 2000, pp. 21–25. Copyright © 2000 The New Republic, Inc. Reproduced by permission.

M anaged care companies work hard to be despised, and they're succeeding. They've offended the public, lost its trust, and recently landed themselves in the Supreme Court. In February 2000, the justices heard the case of Cindy Herdrich, who went to her HMO complaining of abdominal pain. The examining physician found hints of an inflamed appendix. Yet, instead of sending Herdrich for an immediate, full-price ultrasound at the local hospital, the doctor told her to wait eight days—until an appointment became available at an ultrasound facility that offered the HMO a discount. During the wait Herdrich's appendix ruptured, threatening her life. She's already sued the doctor for negligence and won. Now, in her Supreme Court case, Herdrich is arguing that because her HMO gave end-of-the-year bonuses to physicians who held costs down, it violated its fiduciary responsibility to put patients first. Since almost all health insurers now reward cost containment, Herdrich's case could turn managed care upside down, if not outlaw it altogether.

The industry isn't any more popular in the other branches of government. In March 2000, the House and Senate will try to hammer out a compromise version of patients' rights legislation, whose main purpose is to make it easier to sue HMOs. (Some anti-HMO suits are currently barred by a quirk of the law.)[1] Managed care reform also occupies a prominent place in Al Gore's presidential campaign: the vice president has berated Aetna U.S. Healthcare for denying home care to a disabled six-month-old boy in Washington state. Even George W. Bush has begun bragging about a Texas patients' rights law passed on his watch, though he neglects to mention that he opposed it at the time.

What makes the assault on managed care so peculiar is that Americans are healthier than ever. It's one thing for the public to loathe an industry whose performance is declining, but the health care business is losing stature at a time when its performance is improving. By almost all measures, U.S. public health gets better every year. Americans are living longer than ever before, and heart disease, stroke, hyperten-

1. As of September 2000, a congressional compromise had not been reached. However, forty-two states had set up independent boards to review HMO decisions.

sion, AIDS, and most forms of cancer are steadily declining. Almost every U.S. health trend has been positive during the decade of managed care. And, after rising at a frightening pace for most of the 1980s, the cost of health care has stabilized. There are still serious problems with the system—chiefly that 43 million Americans, a staggering 16 percent of the population, have no health insurance. But bashing managed care, as has become so fashionable, doesn't solve that problem. It just distracts us from it.

Managed Care Successfully Controls Costs

The headquarters of Aetna U.S. Healthcare, the nation's largest managed care firm, sits in a suburban office park in Blue Bell, Pennsylvania, near Philadelphia. Inside the complex, company analysts dictate what medical procedures will or will not be paid for, computers scan records to determine which doctors are holding down costs and which are spending freely, and nurse practitioners line the phone banks that patients and doctors must call to authorize treatment. Aetna controls medical care for about 21 million people; about 300,000 physicians, more than a third of the country's doctors, participate in its plans.

This market power makes Aetna remarkably similar to the "regional alliances" that formed the centerpiece of Bill and Hillary Clinton's 1993 health care plan. Under Hillarycare, a few large regional insurance alliances would have used their clout to negotiate discounts with doctors and hospitals. This is exactly what Aetna and all other major managed care firms now do. Over the past five years, the nation's 18 largest for-profit plans have evolved into six—Aetna, United Healthcare, Cigna, Foundation Health Systems, Pacificare, and Wellpoint Health Networks; and, at this writing, Aetna and Wellpoint were talking about a merger.[2] In about half of all states, the five biggest managed care firms now account for at least 50 percent of patients; in 16 states, they account for more than 70 percent. As a result, the vast majority of physicians and clinics, not to mention almost all hospitals,

2. Aetna rejected a takeover offer from Wellpoint Health Networks and the proposed merger did not take place.

must accept managed care to stay in business. About 125 million Americans belong to HMOs or similar plans roughly three-quarters of the non-Medicare population, with the proportion steadily rising. In effect, Clinton's "regional alliance" plan passed—but through the free market rather than through Congress.

And, at least when it comes to cost control, the plan is working. In 1993, health care consumed 13.7 percent of the nation's GDP, and the rate was shooting upward; many projected it would hit 15 or even 18 percent by the year 2000. By 1998, the most recent year for which statistics are available, spending was down to 13.5 percent of GDP. Because runaway medical inflation is a story that didn't happen, the accomplishment has been overlooked. But that does not diminish its significance. If health care expenditures had risen as expected, today this issue would dominate domestic politics. Middle-class Americans would face ruinous increases in insurance premiums, and voters would be livid. Instead, against the best predictions, health care inflation has cooled. Managed care deserves the credit.

Indeed, little-noticed in the coverage of Herdrich's case was the Clinton administration's decision to file a friend-of-the-court brief opposing her position. The White House may bash opponents of the patients' bill of rights legislation before Congress, but it continues to advance the theory of managed care. In one of his final domestic policy initiatives, Clinton recently proposed that Medicare be allowed to steer senior citizens to physicians and hospitals that offer low fees, just as managed care companies like Aetna do. The administration realizes that if Herdrich wins her Supreme Court case, managed care could go down in flames, taking medical cost control along with it—and we'd suddenly be back to a health care "crisis."

Managed Care Controls Cost by Negotiating Discounts

But aren't managed care's cost-control methods excessive? Not necessarily. Many HMOs control costs through "capitation," or paying a fixed amount per year per patient. Physicians endlessly complain that this means they lose money on really sick patients; they rarely add that it also means they come out ahead on healthy customers. All managed care plans negotiate discounts, mainly through "preferred provider organizations" or "independent practice associations" in which patients are steered to physicians or hospitals that agree to lower their rates. Under such pressure, the prevailing obstetrician's fee for prenatal care and normal delivery of a baby in Washington, D.C., to cite one example, has fallen from about $3,000 in 1993 to about $800 today. While few doctors or hospital administrators are happy about the pressure to discount, discounting has hardly made medicine unrewarding. The income of the average U.S. physician has fallen five percent in real-dollar terms since 1993, but, at $164,000 annually, it remains the highest average physician salary in the world.

To be sure, managed care sometimes imposes maddening precertification requirements—maddening to doctors as well as to patients, since, essentially, the new system automatically questions their judgment. Then there is "utilization review"—insurance companies mine files to see whether particular doctors are ordering unneeded tests, allowing patients to spend too many nights in the hospital, or prescribing proprietary drugs when generic would do. "Case managers," usually nurses, may recommend costcutting ideas to the physicians of seriously ill patients who are running up big bills. Finally, managed care firms sometimes reduce costs by brute force—simply refusing to pay some or all of what physicians and hospitals charge and causing financial disaster for patients who assumed their bills would be covered. (The law on this point is elaborate, but health insurers are not always obligated to pay.)

Baffling Rules and Red Tape Contribute to Poor Image

Some managed care techniques are clearly designed to baffle patients and physicians in the hope they will give up and go away. The section of Aetna's website that lists information patients must know to comply with company rules is 60 printed pages long. And the red tape creates inequality: white-collar professionals accustomed to reading fine print can usually pressure their managed care firms to pay for whatever they need, while the less educated are more likely to give up in frustration. These represent real problems, but they don't explain why so many Americans consider managed care a failure.

The Importance of Preventive Care

Preventive care is one of the most important parts of a primary care physician's job. Consistent adherence to a well-conceived preventive services policy can help make a big difference in patients' health—and lives. . . .

Overall, managed care has had a positive effect on the quality and availability of the most common preventive services. Health plans are concerned about preventive care because their accrediting body, the National Center for Quality Assurance, uses the Health Employer Data Information System (HEDIS) to evaluate managed care companies. HEDIS measures include a number of preventive services. Thus, most health plans pay some, if not all, preventive costs. In addition, many managed care companies are reaching out to urge their members to obtain preventive care. Plans also give feedback as to how the physician is doing in providing preventive services.

Charlotte LoBuono, *Patient Care*, November 15, 1999.

Working on this article, I spent weeks negotiating with Aetna for permission to enter its Pennsylvania stronghold and interview the people who set its claim-approval policies and answer its preapproval phone lines. Arranging interviews at Aetna, it turns out, is harder than arranging them at the Pentagon. The company kept scheduling interviews and later canceling them, then finally declared that its officials and preapproval personnel were just so incredibly, astonishingly busy—every single one of them—that no meeting was possible. Aetna, which has a horrible public image, seemed determined to convince me that it deserved it. In this it reflects the managed care industry in general, which has compiled the most spectacular record of negative public relations since the nuclear power industry of the 1970s.

The shame is that if managed care companies were less creepy, they could make a compelling case that their existence serves the public good. HMOs are not some marketing gimmick; they arose as a rational response to the faults of the old pass-along system, in which physicians passed along unlimited invoices and insurers passed along unlimited inflation. Patients may suffer when a test or procedure is not immediately approved, but they can also be harmed by overtreatment—which the old system encouraged by paying doctors and hospitals to run up the bill. It's not necessarily bad to have case managers watching over a doctor's shoulder; they may point out something the doctor has missed. And some aspects of the new order actually make things easier for patients. In many managed care plans, you never have to fill out forms or front the cash before filing for reimbursement; you just flash your card—a convenience previously known only in national health systems.

Advantages like these are rarely discussed, because we have become convinced that what Cindy Herdrich experienced is now the norm—that managed care is responsible mainly for medical horrors. Yet, if that were really the case, public health would be getting worse. Instead, Harry Rosenberg, chief of mortality data for the National Center for Health Statistics, called 1999 "a banner year" for U.S. public health. A new study by economists Kevin Murphy and Robert Topel of the University of Chicago estimates the annual value of the ever-higher U.S. life expectancy at about $2.8 trillion, more than twice what the nation spends on health care. That people are living longer, more productive lives while losing less time to illness and pain, Murphy and Topel suppose, is one reason the economy is so robust.

No Difference in Health Outcomes Between Managed Care and Fee-for-Service Programs

Nor have studies found any association between managed care and those health care problems that persist. Robert Brook, Elizabeth McGlynn, and Mark Schuster, three physicians who specialize in care-quality data, recently completed an extensive study for the Rand Corporation. They concluded that for overall health outcomes, there is no difference between managed care and traditional fee-for-service programs. (Problems like inequity in service between affluent and poor communities, they found, predate managed care.) Most other studies also conclude that managed care has not harmed patient health, though some analysts find that patients do better in nonprofit managed care than in for-profit plans.

Many people assumed managed care would stunt the development of more effective or more humane treatments by driving all medical services toward whatever is cheapest. That has not happened; expensive procedures continue to proliferate. Two decades ago, for example, artificial joints were a rarity; now almost all insurers pay for hip-replacement surgery. Heart bypass surgery is much more frequent than it was a decade ago—extending life, with vigor, even for those who have the operation in their seventies. Traumatic invasive procedures have been replaced by laparoscopic surgeries, done routinely on an outpatient basis with short recovery times. Not that long ago, a middle-aged adult experiencing chronic knee pain would have been informed that joints begin to ache with age, given ibuprofen, and told to live with it. Today, anything from laparoscopic surgery to an artificial knee is likely to be approved by almost any managed care plan, with the result that the pain is removed.

And, stereotypes aside, waiting is rarely a problem under the new system. The reason Herdrich's case drew so much attention is because what happened to her is so unusual; even with cost containment, patients rarely queue. Today, in Canada's national health system, there is a median wait of six weeks to consult a specialist for nonemergency conditions and a median wait of eleven weeks for a nonemergency MRI. Figures for many Western European national health systems are similar. In the United States, waits of more than a few days for nonemergency tests or therapy are almost nonexistent, because—even under managed care—American medicine has far more hospital beds, specialists, and high-tech equipment per capita than national health systems do. Managed care has pressured the specialists and the owners of fancy medical machines to cut prices, but it has not put them out of business. Unless you're one of the uninsured, this is a best-case result.

Managed Care Forces Efficiency

Health has improved at the same time as costs have declined because managed care has forced doctors and hospitals to become more efficient; they may not enjoy this experience, but their increased efficiency serves society. Though many predicted managed care would cause health care rationing, for the insured, at least, there is zero evidence of it. Stories of HMOs denying a class of treatment almost always involve experimental procedures of questionable merit, such as bone-marrow transplants to treat breast cancer, which new studies suggest are worthless. Extremely expensive but proven procedures, such as bypass surgery and organ transplants, are routinely paid for by managed care, not rationed. Kafkaesque nightmares do occur under managed care, but, contrary to conventional wisdom, they are kinks in a basically successful system.

Working out the kinks remains important. But the stampede toward more anti-HMO lawsuits may not be the best course. As often happens in politics, the debate runs behind developments in the field. Responding to patient dismay, several large managed care organizations—including United Healthcare, the number-two insurer nationally, and many of the Blue Shield plans—have recently eliminated most precertification requirements and now allow patients to go directly to specialists without the approval of a "gatekeeper." Assuming United Healthcare's approach proves popular, firms like Aetna will have to either match it or lose business.

Moreover, denied claims appear to be less of a problem now than they were in the early '90s, when the managed care industry was first figuring itself out. Although it took until 2000 for Herdrich's case to reach the Supreme Court, her mistreatment occurred in 1991. Since that time, fears of liability under existing law, predating a congressional patients' bill of rights, have changed the managed care landscape. In 1993, a California HMO lost an $89 million judgment to the estate of a woman named Nelene Fox, who had been denied needed treatment. This and other decisions shook the industry, making the big carriers look more favorably on treatment requests, especially with juries inclined to believe the worst about HMOs. . . .

None of this is to imply that America's health care system is, by any stretch, morally acceptable. In no other Western nation does a larger percentage of the population lack health insurance. Just as managed care is a logical outcome of market forces, so are the uninsured. Insurers have no free-market incentive to seek out customers who have trouble paying their premiums or who suffer from "preexisting" conditions. Employers trying to cut back health benefits are only acting logically, given the way the rules are currently written. The market controls costs, and it pursues quality of care much more effectively than most commentators acknowledge. But the free market will never look after everyone. That is not its incentive structure.

Insuring that everyone is cared for is the natural role of government. . . . Any solution will cost money, though some of the funds will be recovered through better health and higher productivity among those now uninsured. But the good news is that such money is available, in part because managed care helped save it.

Managed care proves that extensive reform of the medical system, often deemed impossible, can actually happen quickly and with success.

"Managed care stepped in—indeed, it arrived in an ambulance answering a 911 call from ratepayers."

Managed Care Is Necessary to Control Health Care Costs

Thomas W. Hazlett

Managed care provides high-quality, low-cost medical care to consumers, Thomas W. Hazlett argues in the following viewpoint. Doctors who complain that they can not properly treat patients under managed care are really just complaining about a decrease in their status and income, he contends. Moreover, Hazlett maintains that patients report high levels of satisfaction with managed care. Thomas W. Hazlett is an economist at the University of California at Davis and a resident scholar at the Enterprise Institute for Public Policy Research.

As you read, consider the following questions:
1. According to the author, who has been more successful in making sure most people have access to health care?
2. What does Hazlett say was the annual medical cost inflation in the peak year of 1991?
3. According to Hazlett, how do most Americans rate their HMOs relative to traditional health insurance?

Thomas W. Hazlett, "HMO Phobia: Quack Remedies for the Health Care 'Crisis,'" *Reason*, vol. 30, February 1999, pp. 74–75. Copyright © 1999 by Reason Foundation, 3415 S. Sepulveda Blvd., Suite 400, Los Angeles, CA 90034, www.reason.com. Reproduced with permission.

D r. Ken Smith has a mission: to destroy the HMO system which today enrolls 85 percent of insured Americans. The Boston-based physician's reasons are simple and
humane: "We are for patients, not profits." And his disgust
is real: "How dare somebody in some board room in Con-
necticut decide what I'm worth, and on a whim decide that
my worth should be reduced?"

The elements of the current crusade against managed care
combine the front-page horror story of the access-denied
victim with the political clout of a network of influential mil-
lionaires. In swank country clubs all across the land, high-
powered attorneys are burying the hatchet with prosperous
physicians, getting beyond that little multibillion-dollar spat
over medical malpractice. Now they're toasting martinis and
swearing litigation against the common enemy: HMOs that
clamp down on medical costs.

It may shock the good Dr. Smith, but many of the common folk are quite used to having distant big shots in far-
away boardrooms establish the price for their labor. And as
for the purity of spirit to which Smith appeals, we do appreciate the thought. But it's best to avoid any kind of competition regarding who's been more successful in bringing health
care to the masses, the typical HMO shareholder vs. the typical M.D. After all, who is more likely to be recreating out
on the golf course Wednesday afternoon?

Managed Care Controls Costs

The health care market is tricky, and the shadow under
which all discussion takes place is the cost explosion tied to
third-party payments. When Dr. Smith was perfectly free to
prescribe for "his" patient and push the costs onto others—well, that was the Golden Age for doctors. And, coin-
cidentally, 9.9 percent annual medical cost inflation (just to
pick the peak year, 1991) for the rest of us.

Managed care stepped in—indeed, it arrived in an ambulance answering a 911 call from ratepayers. HMOs had a
tough job to do, teaching lots of doctors with egos the size of
Smith's that there ain't no such thing as a free surgical procedure. They have yet to succeed; a group Smith has helped to
organize, The Ad Hoc Committee to Defend Health Care,

protests the "HMO bean counters" and advocates a single-payer system.

The reality is that the rationing that accompanies state-run systems makes the HMOs look like big spenders. That's not because the government hires better "bean counters." Quite the reverse—the beans sort of just disappear. And then it's, "Sorry, you'll just have to wait on that heart bypass until some more beans turn up."

Managed Care Continues to Evolve

"The story of managed care is a story of evolution. Managed care is truly embarking on a new stage in its life cycle," Karen Ignagni, president of the American Association of Health Plans told *MANAGED HEALTHCARE.* "While we have made progress in the area of preventive care, coordinated care and disease management, the emergence of new technology to support these initiatives will allow us to do even more in the future. As a practical matter, the industry has impacted the dynamics of cost and quality far more than any alternative approaches in medical history. . . . The combination of new technology and classic disease management principles has created a true sense of collaboration between providers and payers in an industry that was once very contentious."

Ian R. Lazarus, *Managed Healthcare,* October 2000.

Marc Roberts, a Harvard economist specializing in health care markets, claims that the doctors' real aim is "to regain status, power and income that they lost in this for-profit industry," and that holding the patient's welfare out as a bargaining chip is a smart stratagem. "They wouldn't gain any support if they stood up and said, 'Instead of making $300,000, I now make $200,000, and you should all feel sorry for me.'" The blunt fact is that letting doctors run up medical tabs resulted in runaway expenditures, stealing money from the pockets of wage earners, who ultimately pay in the form of reduced take-home.

Unaffordability is itself a cause of illness, as it puts more Americans outside the health insurance system altogether, lessening their access to regular checkups and preventive medicine. Instead, they increasingly resort to visits to crowded hospital emergency rooms. Treatment there is inefficiently administered—and quietly tacked onto the bills of paying customers, further driving up costs and pushing more working people out.

Consumers Must Pay for Choices

As consumers, many of us prefer plans which offer a wide range of choice among doctor and treatments. But to receive the benefits from that high-cost deal, we do—and should— pay more via higher premiums and lower reimbursements. Government surely has a role to play enforcing contracts with insurers who attempt to renege and as a smart shopper purchasing large volumes of health care directly. (My understanding is that neither courts nor Medicare and Medicaid are as yet perfectly administered.)

The pressure to realistically assess the cost-benefit trade-offs in medical care should be welcomed by those outside the fashionable salons where "for-profit" medicine is profitably denounced. In fact, the overwhelming majority of Americans find their HMOs good to excellent, and most rate them as superior to traditional health insurance on the value/dollar scale.

That's a state of affairs that the HMO reformers aim to change. Stuart Altman, professor of health policy at Brandeis University, notes: "The more we reduce the power of managed care to control spending by restricting services, the more we are going to take [away] the pressure of providers to constrain spending."

That's what doctors want, that's why lawyers will sue, and that's the reason Congress will legislate. But don't feel left out—you'll get the bill.

"Patients consume medical services with little regard for cost when someone else is paying for them."

Managed Care Is Not Necessary to Control Health Care Costs

Larry Van Heerden

In the following viewpoint, Larry Van Heerden contends that the managed care system is unnecessary and expensive. Because managed care requires only a token copayment, it removes the patient's incentive to economize, Van Heerden argues. In addition, he maintains that because managed care measures the effectiveness of health care delivery, not the effectiveness of individual physicians, HMOs make it impossible for patients to choose the best doctor for their health care dollar. Larry Van Heerden is the author of the website Free Market Medicine.

As you read, consider the following questions:
1. According to Larry Van Heerden, what is the central tenet of managed care?
2. How should health care be treated, according to the author?
3. In Van Heerden's opinion, what should doctors be able to do if their patients do not comply with treatment plans?

Larry Van Heerden, "Free-Market Medicine," *Ideas on Liberty*, August 2002, pp. 42–47. Copyright © 2002 by *Ideas on Liberty*. Reproduced by permission.

The health-care system in the United States is beset by problems. After years of feeling shortchanged by managed care, doctors and hospitals are demanding and getting greater compensation; the elderly (under Medicare) have no prescription coverage; and many people find health insurance of any kind unaffordable. Managed care, which was hailed as the answer to spiraling costs, is under legislative and legal assault, while health-care costs are rising at double-digit rates. Proposed solutions range from a Canadian-style single-payer system to medical savings accounts to staying the course with managed care. . . .

How Managed Care Failed

Managed care, which came into prominence in the 1990s, was initially successful at holding down health-care costs. However, doctors, hospitals, and patients were soon fighting back, and the inherent weaknesses of third-party control were revealed: By requiring patients to pay no more than a token copayment, managed care removes the incentive to economize and undermines patient control of health-care encounters. The central tenet of managed care is that consumers are ill-equipped to deal directly with health-care providers; managed-care organizations must act as intermediaries, handling the complexities of medical payment and quality assessment, leaving consumers to make their wishes known by choosing from a list of rival health plans provided by their employers. This is an anemic form of competition, which is as effective in securing cost-effective health care as a passenger would be in arriving at his destination by telling a blindfolded driver when to step on the accelerator, hit the brake, or turn the steering wheel. To achieve the goal of cost-effective care, consumers need to choose at the level of the individual provider and medical procedure, and face both the costs and benefits of their choices.

A more fundamental problem with managed care is that many medical decisions fall into a gray area where definitive scientific judgment cannot be rendered for individual cases. This gray area is the subject of a tug of war between patients and managed-care administrators. Patients, many of whom are being treated for diseases partly of their own making, want no expense to be spared in their treatment, since some-one else is footing the bill. Managed-care organizations, on the other hand, make money (or stay solvent) by limiting the amount of care rendered to subscribers. This gray area is large enough to make the difference between financial success and failure for the organizations and large enough to give pa-tients who are denied care plenty of ammunition when seek-ing legislative and legal action against those organizations.

Single-Payer System Is Filled with Problems

A Canadian-style single-payer health care system is nothing more than a massive managed-care arrangement with gov-ernment bureaucrats in control and without a meaningful ap-peals process for care denied or delayed. The same problems inherent in private managed care arise in a government-run system. Moreover, as a rule, government programs cannot satisfy consumer demand. Since all goods and services are fi-nite and require human effort to produce, rationing is un-avoidable. Only the method of rationing is subject to choice. The free market rations on the basis of income; the method of rationing is the familiar pricing system. When this system is circumvented by the government to provide a "free" good or service, all constraints on demand are removed, making inevitable the explicit rationing of supply by some govern-ment authority or the disappearance of the good or service altogether. Regarding universal access to health care, it should be noted that before government intervention in the health-care system, a variety of private organizations pro-vided free medical care to the poor.

Medical Savings Accounts Are Controlled by Individuals

Medical savings account (MSA) health plans were intro-duced at the federal level as a demonstration project in 1996. The central feature of these employer-provided plans is a savings account controlled by the insured individual and used to pay for routine health care. An accompanying low-cost catastrophic insurance policy covers health-care ex-penses that exceed the high yearly deductible. MSA plans enjoy the same tax advantage as other employer-provided health insurance. Although unspent MSA funds roll over from year to year, they can only be spent on health care.

The high deductible associated with MSA health plans leads to substantial savings in administrative costs because many low-dollar claims for routine medical care are never filed. In addition, having patients spending their own money on health care makes them more prudent consumers, which means less spending on unnecessary health care services.

However, MSA health plans have drawbacks. They perpetuate the income tax distortion of health-care spending and are subject to legislative manipulation: Under current law, MSA plans are hamstrung by limited availability and growth, unnecessary complexity, and design features that put them at a disadvantage in the marketplace. Finally, MSA critics argue that the very idea of government direction or control of consumer spending is inimical to a free market.

How a Market-Driven Solution Works

The solution to the problems discussed above is to treat health care more like other products and services. This means repealing all tax exemptions for health insurance and health-care spending, enacting a compensating tax cut unrelated to individual health-care consumption, eliminating all health-insurance mandates and other regulation, and letting the market sort things out.

The market would probably respond to such deregulation the same way it did before government intervened in health care: As early as the 1940s commercial insurers included deductibles and copayments in their sickness insurance offerings and excluded many elective treatments from coverage, all in an effort to restrain demand for unnecessary and costly medical services. Commercial insurers also used actuarial risks to calculate premium payments and paid individual subscribers, instead of hospitals. Giving patients a substantial financial stake in the cost of their care will make them interested in the cost-effectiveness of that care.

A second part of a market-driven solution would likely be giving patients access to information comparing the performance of competing physicians, just as consumer magazines provide information on competing products. To do this, independent organizations might determine what physicians accomplish in a clinical setting by measuring the health status of patients before and after treatment. To be cost-effective, such measurement would probably make use of electronic medical records.

The Individual Must Take the Lead

Managed care embodies an effort by employers, insurers, and some physician organizations to establish priorities, balance competing goals, and decide who should get what from the US health care system. After a turbulent decade of trial and error, that experiment can be characterized as a partial economic success and total political failure. The strategy of giving with one hand while taking away with the other, of offering consumers comprehensive benefits while restricting access through utilization review, obfuscates the workings of the system, undermines trust between patients and physicians, and has infuriated everyone involved.

The protagonists of the managed care system now are in full retreat, broadening panels, removing restrictions, reverting to fee-for-service, and generally getting out from between consumers and the services they want to consume. The retreat from managed care promotes access but also removes the brakes on health care cost inflation. The individual consumer and patient is the last candidate for the difficult but necessary role of balancing resources and expectations.

James C. Robinson, *Journal of the American Medical Association*, May 21, 2001.

Employees on expense accounts spend much more freely than when making purchases with their own hard-earned money. Similarly, patients consume medical services with little regard for cost when someone else is paying for them. In a climate of unnecessary medical care, preventable disease, and medical uncertainty, insulating consumers from the cost of choices they or their doctors make guarantees inefficiency and runaway costs.

Cost-Sharing Reduces Use of Medical Services

Cost-sharing refers to the requirement that patients bear a significant share of the cost of all medical care rendered in their behalf. It does not refer to paying insurance premiums (which do nothing to constrain health-care consumption).

The RAND health-insurance experiment showed that patients who have to pay for part of their care cut back substantially on the use of medical services. While the market will figure out the right mix of deductibles and copayments, it seems likely that as an individual's yearly health-care expenses rise, his out-of-pocket share of new health-care expenditures will decline. However, from an economic point of view, it would be optimal if no one's out-of-pocket share of medical expenses ever dropped to zero, giving every consumer a stake in the cost of every medical visit, test, procedure, hospitalization, or prescription drug he consumes. An immediate effect of such cost-sharing would be to give physicians a newly found interest in cost control for the benefit of their patients and as a means to attract business. . . .

In an attempt to control costs, managed-care organizations have been measuring the process of health-care delivery, rather than identifying physicians who keep their patients healthy. In a newly deregulated market, one can imagine managed-care organizations dropping their review and oversight functions in favor of collecting and disseminating (for a fee) information on the performance of physicians (and eventually hospitals). If such a service were to periodically measure a patient's health status during the course of treatment, the change in these measurements, collected for a sufficient number of patients (and adjusted for severity of illness, co-morbidity, and patient demographics), could be used to measure doctors based on the results they achieve in their patients.

Assessing outcomes is appealing because of its narrow focus: As long as a patient's health status can be objectively measured, none of the intervening steps that are part of medical treatment need be evaluated. Concern about the number and type of tests performed, improper use of high-tech equipment, medications prescribed, or the appropriateness of the treatment chosen would be superfluous. Poor choices by a physician in such matters would either be reflected in higher costs or worse outcomes than those of other physicians.

For preventive medicine and most chronic diseases the performance of physicians is inextricably linked to patient compliance and cooperation. As a result, the performance of physician and patient would probably have to be measured jointly. Nonetheless, in the context of a system controlled by any third party, measuring a physician based on the behavior of his patients would likely be unacceptable to the marketplace.

However, in a health-care system that includes patient cost-sharing, measuring the performance of physician and patient jointly makes sense. No third-party coercion would be needed; a patient's financial stake in the cost of care would serve as a necessary and sufficient constraint on his behavior. . . .

Doctors who felt certain patients weren't living up to their end of the bargain (regarding compliance with treatment plans) would be free to refer them elsewhere. Thus the goals of physician and patient would be in alignment.

Indicators to be measured would probably be those known to be closely related to good health and closely related in time to physician intervention. Examples of possible indicators are cholesterol levels, blood pressure, blood-glucose levels, and patient satisfaction.

The Government Would Ensure Privacy

The government would play an important role in establishing and enforcing a patient's right to control his medical information. Beyond that, patient privacy would be protected because the measurement system would not need identifying information.

The health-care market has failed to produce high-quality, low-cost medicine for two reasons: Consumers are insulated from the cost of medical care by third-party payers, and information on the performance of competing physicians is not available. Fixing the incentives and providing consumers with physician performance data will cause unnecessary surgery to decline, physician performance to improve, disease prevention to increase, and health-care efficiency to rise.

> *"In the Roper and ABC surveys, those in managed care were more satisfied than were those in traditional arrangements with costs."*

Most Patients Are Satisfied with Managed Care

Karlyn Bowman

In the following viewpoint, Karlyn Bowman uses data from respected national polls to argue that most managed care patients are satisfied with their health care. In fact, she maintains, these polls indicate there is little difference in satisfaction between those in managed-care arrangements and those in traditional fee-for-service plans. She contends that Americans' dislike for big bureaucracies and biased media coverage are responsible for the negative image of HMOs. Karlyn Bowman is a writer and resident fellow at the American Enterprise Institute for Public Policy Research.

As you read, consider the following questions:
1. According to the author, what did Charlton Research show was the most important health care problem?
2. In Bowman's opinion, what role do most Americans feel that the federal government should play in health plan or insurance management?
3. What does Bowman say is responsible for managed care's negative image?

Karlyn Bowman, "Is Managed Health Care Unpopular?" *AEI on the Issues*, June 1998. Copyright © 1998 by American Enterprise Institute for Public Policy Research. Reproduced by permission.

The authoritative *National Journal* gives voice to conventional wisdom when it claims that "no one doubts that so-called patient protection bills are highly popular." Anecdotal evidence of frustration and irritation with managed care and of horror stories about botched care makes it seem almost pointless to argue with the journal's description of a "public outcry." But sometimes the conventional wisdom is wrong, or at least seriously misleading. Anyone who has reviewed carefully what people with coverage are saying about their care comes away with a much different impression.

People in traditional fee-for-service care are generally more satisfied than are those in managed-care arrangements. But differences are small, and there is little evidence of widespread unhappiness in either group. A Roper Starch Worldwide survey found that 80 percent of managed-care patients in 1996 were satisfied with the quality of their care, as were 82 percent in fee-for-service care; 77 percent in managed care were satisfied with the availability of medical care when they needed it, as were 79 percent in traditional care. In 1997, ABC News found 83 percent of patients in health maintenance organizations and 87 percent in traditional arrangements satisfied with their ability to get a doctor's appointment, and 81 percent in HMOs and 90 percent in traditional care satisfied with their ability to see top-quality specialists. In the eight areas that ABC explored, satisfaction levels were similar.

Moreover, in the ABC poll, 78 percent of those in traditional arrangements said that they would recommend their plan. So did 79 percent of those in HMOs. This is hardly evidence of widespread dissatisfaction.

The cost of health care, long a worry to people, remains a big concern. When Charlton Research asked respondents to name the country's most important health-care problem, 60 percent mentioned cost and, separately, affordability. Cost swamped other problems, such as lack of choice in insurance plans and restriction on choice of doctors.

In the Roper and ABC surveys, those in managed care were *more* satisfied than were those in traditional arrangements with costs. Sixty-two percent of the former and 53 percent of the latter told Roper that their costs were reasonable. Seventy-nine percent in HMOs and 65 percent in traditional arrangements in the ABC survey said that they were satisfied with their costs.

Managed Care Is Good for the Sick

The data do not support the notion that managed care is good for those who are healthy and bad for the sick. One-third of respondents told ABC that they or someone in their family had had a serious illness or injury while under their current plan. Of those, 93 percent in traditional arrangements said that they were satisfied with the medical care they or their families had received, but so were 88 percent in HMOs. Eighty-six percent with traditional care and 84 percent of those in HMOs reported being satisfied with their insurance coverage during this time. Louis Harris and Harvard University looked at the experiences of those with a "higher burden of illness." They reported that the "vast majority of these people are satisfied with many aspects of their health care regardless of the type of health plan they have." On fifteen of sixty-six items, the researchers found significant differences between limited-choice managed care and fee-for-service care. Twenty-two percent of the sick in managed care and 13 percent in fee-for-service care, for example, reported major or minor problems in getting treatment that they and their doctors deemed necessary. The differences were generally of this level and magnitude.

The Role of Government

Americans continue to believe that the federal government has an important role to play in this area. Just 14 percent in a Kaiser Family Foundation/Harvard University survey said that very little or no government regulation was needed for health plans or health insurance. But the desire for government oversight collides with real concern that government action will increase costs, and also with widespread skepticism about federal government performance. Seventy percent in a Kaiser/Harvard survey said that having a hotline telephone number for people to call when they have problems with their plan was "very important." When the word "government" was added to the word "hotline," the proportion saying "very important" dropped to 43 percent.

HMO Patients Are Pleased

Although the overwhelming majority of people in HMOs are very satisfied with their care, public opinion polls indicate that a majority of the general public feels that HMOs would not provide all the care needed in the event of a serious illness. These attitudes—and the resulting effect they may have on assessments of care—may be driven by anecdotes heard from a friend or read in the press, rather than by personal experience. Thus, a few visible cases where patients do not receive needed care can lead to widespread unfavorable assessments, even if the vast majority of HMO enrollees' own experiences are positive. In fact, since only one half of one percent of HMO enrollees report not being able to see a specialist as a reason for not receiving or having to delay needed care, the public appears to view the risk of being denied access to a specialist for needed care as being greater in an HMO than is likely the case.

James D. Reschovsky et al., Center for Studying Health System Change, Issue Brief 28, March 2000.

Three times in the years 1996 through 1998, Kaiser/Harvard posed these statements: "Some people say that new government regulation is needed to protect consumers from being treated unfairly and not getting the care they should from managed-care plans. Others say this additional regulation isn't worth the cost because it would raise the cost of health insurance too much for everyone." In December 1997, the public split 44 percent in favor of new regulation, 47 percent opposed. When Kaiser/Harvard probed people's reactions to elements in the consumer bill of rights, they found substantial support for them—in the abstract. But when they followed up, asking people whether they would still favor each proposal even if it resulted in an increase in premium costs, or if the measure would get the federal government more involved, or if it would result in employers dropping coverage, the decline in support was dramatic in each area.

In another question, 72 percent favored legislation to protect health-care consumers. But just 43 percent in this Kaiser/Harvard survey said that they would support it if their premium increase were $1–$5 per month. Only 28 percent would support a $15–$20 per month increase. . . .

Positive Personal Experience Versus Negative Media Coverage

So what explains the impression of *National Journal* reporters and others that managed care is unpopular? Start with the fact that Americans don't like big bureaucracies—neither President Bill Clinton's 1993 plan nor managed-care conglomerates. Add to that the fact that change is always unsettling, and probably more so in an area as sensitive as health care, where most of us consider ourselves unsophisticated. Media coverage plays a role, too. The Kaiser Family Foundation looked at coverage of managed care between 1990 and 1997 and pronounced it neutral. But when they looked specifically at broadcast news (most Americans get their news from television), coverage was overwhelmingly negative. Beyond this, most of us know someone who has had a bad or irritating experience with managed care, and the horror stories are genuinely troubling. These factors explain why surveys about managed care—as opposed to the more relevant and authentic questions about personal experience—often produce negative results.

None of this is to say that some reforms aren't necessary and desirable. But if we get the diagnosis wrong, the cure won't work.

> "Middle-class families who once feared that government bureaucrats might micro-manage their health care were now finding that insurance company bureaucrats were doing the same thing."

Most Patients Are Not Satisfied with Managed Care

Andrew Phillips

In the following viewpoint, Andrew Phillips argues that with the advent of Health Maintenance Organizations (HMOs), middle-class Americans have started to worry about being denied the health care they need. He maintains that while managed care helps control health-care costs, it limits patients' choices in doctors and applies stricter rules for the types of treatment allowed. According to Phillips, patients' fears about HMOs have increased as the number of "horror stories" about poor managed care proliferate. Andrew Phillips is a staff writer for *Maclean's*.

As you read, consider the following questions:

1. In Phillips's opinion, managed care takes crucial health care decisions away from doctors and turns them over to whom?
2. Which country has the highest health care costs in the industrialized world, according to Phillips?
3. What is targeted by the anti-HMO campaign, according to the author?

Andrew Phillips, "Mismanaged Care: Americans Are Angry About Their Health Care," *Maclean's*, vol. 111, July 20, 1998, p. 20. Copyright © 1998 Maclean Hunter Canadian Publishing Ltd. Reproduced by permission.

Paul Ruskin admits it: he's obsessed. "I'm compelled to keep fighting," he says. "Sometimes I wish I could stop." For a few hours every week for almost three years, through icy winter days and the sweaty heat of a Maryland summer, Ruskin, 53, has paced outside a hospital run by the health insurance company he believes bungled his wife's medical care, leaving her with permanently impaired vision. "Kaiser misdiagnosed my wife's brain tumor for four years—why?" reads the yellow placard he carries.

It has been a lonely fight. The company, Kaiser Permanente, is one of the biggest private health insurers in the United States, and it denies that it mishandled care for Ruskin's wife of 33 years, Jill. "It's David against Goliath," he says as he marches up and down. These days, though, Ruskin's complaints are being echoed across the land. Americans are increasingly angry about the restrictions on medical treatment imposed by so-called managed-care organizations like Kaiser. Crucial decisions about health care, goes the common refrain, are being taken out of the hands of doctors and turned over to insurance company accountants. Politicians, their eyes fixed on 1998 midterm elections, have jumped on the issue. Democrats and Republicans alike are pushing legislation to enforce "patients' rights" against hard-hearted insurers. In one TV ad that sums up the new mood, a Democratic candidate for governor of Georgia, Roy Barnes, fires off this line: "If you can choose who changes the oil in your car, you should be able to choose who delivers your baby."

The last time health care topped the U.S. political agenda was 1993, when President Bill Clinton proposed a massive program to give more Americans access to medical insurance. Health costs were soaring and millions of Americans could not afford care. The insurance industry successfully portrayed so-called Clintoncare as a manoeuvre by government bureaucrats to take choice away from patients. A $22-million industry ad campaign featuring Harry and Louise, a fictional middle-class couple, aired those anxieties. "They choose," mused Harry, and Louise responded: "We lose." Clinton's plan died in 1994.

The 1998 version of Harry and Louise is Carol, the waitress portrayed by actress Helen Hunt in the movie *As Good as It Gets*. Carol's son suffers from asthma, and when she learns that her health maintenance organization, or HMO, has denied him proper care, she lets loose a string of epithets that had U.S. movie audiences cheering. Politicians noticed, and acted accordingly. Clinton announced his support for a patients' rights bill in his state of the union address in January 1998. Republicans, traditionally skeptical of government fixes and reliant on campaign funds from the health industry, were slower to react. But in late June, they, too, took up the cause. Both parties support giving patients more information about their health plans, greater ability to appeal when they are denied care, and guaranteed access to emergency rooms. The Democrats, though, would go further, and allow patients to sue health plans for improperly denying them treatment.

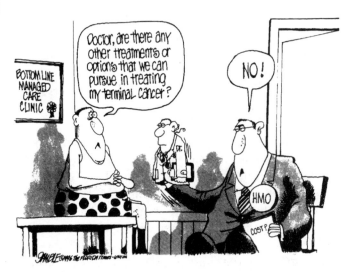

Gamble. © 1996 by *The Florida-Times Union*. Reprinted by permission of Ed Gamble.

What changed between 1993 and 1998? Even though Clinton's plan was defeated, the reasons that inspired it remained. Health costs were rising far faster than inflation. They ate up some 13 percent of the U.S. economy in 1992, and Washington forecast a rise to 18 percent by 2000. Employers, who pay most of the cost of Americans' medical care, were determined to reverse the trend. They transferred more and more of their employees from traditional coverage, where doctors simply bill insurance companies for treatment, to managed-care plans like HMOs, which usually receive a fixed annual fee for each patient they cover. However, patients often must go to doctors chosen by the insurance company, and there are far stricter rules on what kind of treatment is allowed. Some 160 million Americans are now covered by managed care, compared with just 90 million as recently as 1990.

The move worked. In 1996, the growth in health-care spending hit a 37-year low. U.S. doctors' earnings stagnated, at an average of $280,000 a year. Health care still consumes about 13 percent of U.S. economic output—far higher than the 9.6 percent in Canada and the highest in the industrialized world, but considerably lower than had been projected. But the human cost mounted. Middle-class families who once feared that government bureaucrats might micromanage their health care were now finding that insurance company bureaucrats were doing the same thing. "HMO horror stories" became a staple of political discourse.

HMO Horror Stories Abound

Robert Raible, a health-care activist in Washington, has compiled more than 200 such cases. They include a California man who was discharged from hospital four days after receiving a heart transplant because his HMO would not pay for additional hospital care; he soon died. An HMO in Atlanta told a mother to take her six-month-old son with a high fever to one of its clinics 60 km away rather than to a closer hospital, by the time he arrived, he was in cardiac arrest. And a newborn baby in New York City died after he was discharged from hospital after the one day mandated by his parents' HMO—even though his mother voiced concern about his health.

Paul Ruskin's tale is similar. He says his wife, who is 54, went to the doctor assigned to her by Kaiser Permanente in 1987, after an optometrist became concerned about pressure building in her eye. She was diagnosed with glaucoma, and was treated with eyedrops for four years. Eventually, as her vision deteriorated, Jill Ruskin sought treatment elsewhere and a new doctor used a CAT scan to discover that she had a slow-growing benign tumor in her brain. It was removed in 1993. She recovered sufficiently to continue her job as an accountant at a nursing home in suburban Washington, but suffers from impaired vision. Paul Ruskin believes that Kaiser failed to perform a CAT scan or refer Jill to other specialists because its doctors are given financial incentives to limit treatment—something the company denies. He got nowhere in trying to get a settlement out of Kaiser, so he began picketing. "They'll never see the end of this case," he vows.

The irony is that many health-care reformers have advocated managed care as a way of improving Americans' health. Instead of rewarding doctors only when they patch up sick people, went the argument, managed-care companies have an incentive to keep their patients healthy through prevention programs. Even the anti-HMO diatribe in *As Good as It Gets*, though entertaining, may be misleading: HMOs have actually pioneered programs to keep childhood asthma under control. And independent experts rate Kaiser Permanente as one of the best HMOs.

The Insured Middle Class Still Worries

But the populist appeal of attacking managed care is irresistible for many politicians. Clinton's 1993 health-care plan focused on the 37 million Americans who had no medical insurance. That number has jumped to 41 million since then, but the anti-HMO campaign targets the anxieties of the middle-class majority who have insurance, but worry they may still be denied the care they need. "This is an everybody issue," says Democratic political consultant Doc Sweitzer, who has crafted TV ads for congressional candidates aiming to win in November 1998 by bashing insurance companies. The industry, though, is not taking it lying down. In true American political fashion, its response has been quick: a multimillion-dollar TV campaign of its own.

Periodical Bibliography

The following articles have been selected to supplement the diverse views presented in this chapter.

American Medical News	"More Patients Unhappy with Managed Care," June 14, 1999.
Chain Drug Review	"Many Customers Unhappy with Managed Care Plans," August 30, 1999.
Richard A. Epstein	"Managed Care Under Siege," *Journal of Medicine and Philosophy*, October 1999.
Debra S. Feldman, Dennis H. Novack, and Edward Gracely	"Effects of Managed Care on Physician-Patient Relationships, Quality of Care, and the Ethical Practice of Medicine: A Physician Survey," *Archives of Internal Medicine*, August 10, 1998.
Roger Feldman	"The Ability of Managed Care to Control Health Care Costs: How Much Is Enough?" *Journal of Health Care Finance*, Spring 2000.
Marsha Gold	"The Changing U.S. Health Care System: Challenges for Responsible Public Policy," *Milbank Quarterly*, Spring 1999.
Julie A. Jacob	"Managed Image," *American Medical News*, December 6, 1999.
George Khushf	"The Case for Managed Care: Reappraising Medical and Socio-Political Ideals," *Journal of Medicine and Philosophy*, October 1999.
Jonathan R. Laing	"Can Managed Care Be Saved? The Free Market Is Transforming America's Health Care System in Far More Efficient Ways than Hillary Clinton Could Ever Dream," *Barron's*, May 15, 2000.
Norra Macready	"Heroic Measures Needed to Save Managed Care," *Internal Medicine News*, November 1, 2001.
Medicine and Health	"MCOs Get Good Ratings, Especially from Medicare Beneficiaries," October 29, 2001.
Modern Physician	"Matter of Trust," October 2001.
Holcomb B. Nobel	"Public Health Groups Debate Managed Care," *New York Times*, November 24, 1998.
Public Health Reports	"Providers, Health Plans Clash over Patient Care," November 1999.
William M. Sullivan	"What Is Left of Professionalism After Managed Care," *The Hastings Center Report*, March 1999.

CHAPTER 3

How Can the Problem of Uninsured Americans Be Solved?

Chapter Preface

There is a place for providers, a place for consumers, a place for insurers, a place for government programs—but over 40 million uninsured Americans wonder if there is also a place for charity in the U.S. health care system of the twenty-first century. Some experts argue that the passage of Medicare and Medicaid in 1965 made doctors' "charity cases" unnecessary, while others maintain that the managed care revolution of the 1970s made them impossible. The advent of Medicare, which gave health care coverage to all Americans over sixty-five, and Medicaid, which provided health care to low-income individuals, meant that doctors, hospitals, and other providers would be paid for services they might have previously rendered without cost. Further, studies done in 1996–1997 and again in 1998–1999 by Marie C. Reed, Peter J. Cunningham, and Jeffery Stoddard at the Center for Studying Health System Change (HSC), suggest that the cost savings generated by managed care have come at the expense of doctors' ability to provide for the uninsured.

The authors of the HSC study show that the number of physicians providing charity care dropped from 76 percent in 1997 to 72 percent in 1999, although the number of hours of care provided by each participating physician (11.1 per month) remained constant. Moreover, while the total number of practicing physicians increased during the survey years from 347,000 to 363,000, the number providing care to the indigent did not.

As Scott Morris, a physician who provides health care for the working poor (those who earn too much to be covered by Medicaid and cannot afford other health insurance) put it, "The safety net that we have relied on to serve them now has many gaping holes." He claims that prior to 1965, fully one-third of every doctor's practice was expected to be charity care. Doctors in private practice staffed teaching hospitals and were expected to spend at least one day a week in the charity clinic. Times have changed, however, according to Morris. He writes: "When asked about our commitment to care for all patients who need our skills, too many of us, along with hospitals, have confused bad debt with true charity care. There are now physicians younger than forty years who have never treated a patient knowing up front that he or she will not get paid. This would never have been the case 30 years ago." Morris believes that each physician has a moral imperative to include the uninsured as "a significant part" of his or her practice—simply because it is the right thing to do.

As the charity care safety net grows more tattered, increased job layoffs and economic uncertainty combined with large increases in insurance premiums, deductibles, and co-payments increase the likelihood that more people will become uninsured or underinsured and will not have access to the health care they need, contend the authors of the HSC study.

However, Carol K. Kane of the American Medical Association's (AMA) Center for Health Policy Research, concedes that although the charity care safety net is a bit strained, it is still strong and secure. She points to a study by the American Medical Association's Socioeconomic Monitoring System (SMS) that surveyed physicians in 1988, 1994, and 1999, and asked them how many hours of free or reduced fee care they provided in their most recent complete week of practice. In 1988, 62 percent of physicians provided charity care (6.6 hours per week); in 1994, more doctors, 67.7 percent, provided more hours of care (7.2 hours) per week. In 1999, the number of doctors tending to charity cases dropped to 64.6 percent, but the hours they spent each week (8.8) increased. Kane insists that tabulation of the SMS data, combined with national estimates of the physician population from the AMA Masterfile, show that the number of physicians providing charity care has actually increased during the years surveyed. She maintains, "Our data show that physician commitment to charity care remains strong."

Many doctors believe that charity care must remain an essential element of the U.S. health care system and the moral responsibility of physicians. In this chapter, authors debate the best solutions for the problem of uninsured Americans. Strengthening the charity care safety net might help many of the nation's poor.

"It is time to rescue the 39 million Americans who are forced to seek care within the system of no-system."

Universal Health Care Is the Best Solution for Uninsured Americans

Robert L. Ferrer

In the following viewpoint, Robert L. Ferrer argues that America's lack of a national health care system has created an institutionalized system of exclusion for those too poor to afford medical insurance. The author maintains that as this "system of no-system" becomes more firmly entrenched, the few resources locally available to poor patients will become even more fragmented and difficult to access. A universal health care system, he contends, is the only way to provide for the 39 million uninsured Americans suffering without proper health care. Robert L. Ferrer is a physician at a county hospital in San Antonio, Texas.

As you read, consider the following questions:

1. According to Ferrer, why do patients in his clinic rarely complain about long waits?
2. In the author's opinion, why are the failures of the safety net he provides not random accidents?
3. What does Ferrer list as the most important example illustrating the failure of the system of no-system?

My waiting room is bigger than yours. It seats 228 and by mid-afternoon it is usually packed. On a good day patients will wait two to three hours to see me or one of the other clinicians who work here. On a bad day the wait can reach five or six hours. Not as many patients complain as you might think. Almost all are uninsured, and they have nowhere else to go. Our "acute care" clinic is a large county-hospital walk-in clinic—the portal of entry to the public health care system in a county in which 360,000 of the 1.3 million inhabitants are uninsured. The numbers are alarming, but the stories underlying them are even worse.

The Uninsured Suffer Most

1. A woman with flank pain, dysuria, and a temperature of 103 who had been seen in a local emergency department (ED) the previous night. She was given some type of injection for pain and sent home. No tests had been done. Results of urinalysis done in our office confirmed pyelonephritis.

2. A man with a sore throat who had spent the previous night in our hospital's ED and left after waiting more than 16 hours to be seen. He had a peritonsillar abscess and needed the care of an otolaryngologist, so we sent him back to the ED. This time he went with a diagnosis.

3. A man who said that his cardiologist sent him to our clinic for "blood pressure medication and a pacemaker." He had fainted during a recent treadmill examination at the cardiologist's office. He then lost his health insurance and could no longer be seen there.

4. A man with a large bandage on his hand. Three days earlier, the fourth and fifth fingers of his left hand had been amputated in a chain saw accident and then reattached at another hospital. Because he had no insurance, he was sent to our walk-in clinic for follow-up.

5. A child sent home from school two weeks earlier with "pink eye." The child's school administration would not readmit her without a doctor's note, and her parents needed two weeks to gather the money for a doctor visit so they could obtain the necessary note.

6. A 22-year-old man with dyspnea, a heart rate of 160, and a large globular heart on his chest film. He came to see

us instead of his "usual" physician because he had recently lost his job and his health insurance because of frequent medical absences caused by his lupus.

7. A middle-aged man with severe shoulder pain and a ruptured short head of his biceps. The consultant refused to see him on an expedited basis, explaining, "These people get free care; they should expect to wait."

8. A homeless man who is a heavy drinker with arm pain. He had been seen several weeks earlier at an ED for the same problem and released without treatment. His humerus was grossly angulated, and a fracture was evident on x-ray. Examination of his head revealed a large depressed skull fracture.

9. An HIV-negative man with fever, cough, weight loss, and *Mycobacterium kansasii* growing from his sputum. He had been seen in the county tuberculosis (TB) clinic but was discharged six months earlier when his culture was reported as not *Mycobacterium tuberculosis*. He was told to "see a doctor."

10. A man in his early 20s with a worsening dental infection who was unable to afford a dentist. He finally saw a physician who prescribed an antibiotic, but the patient was unable to pay for the prescription. He presented to our clinic with sepsis and spread of the infection to his mediastinum. He died soon after admission.

I wish this was a top-ten list of lamentable stories, but it is not. The egregious is commonplace in our setting. My colleagues and I are part of what is widely known as the health care "safety net" for the uninsured, but to work here is to realize that, for many, the safety net does not provide a soft landing, nor are its failures the random "accidents" implied by the image of missing a net.

In actuality, events such as these are the product of a system, an increasingly coherent system of exclusion that denies care to the uninsured: the system of no-system. The system of no-system's components are the fragmented resources locally available to the uninsured, embedded within the national nonsystem of health care. It is a netherworld of closed doors and shrinking services. The paradox of the system of no-system is that it is becoming increasingly systematized. Unintended consequences of changes in health care organization and financing, positive feedback loops enabled by the nonsystem, and maladaptations to the health care market are solidifying the barriers to care for the uninsured.

Features of the System of No-System

Inversion. In the system of no-system, the relationship between needs and resources is inverted. Services are least available to those who need them most, a situation aptly named the "inverse care law" in 1971 by the English general practitioner Julian Tudor Hart. As Tudor Hart pointed out, the inverse care law is exacerbated by a market distribution of medical care because poor people suffer the highest levels of disease and distress but offer the least financial incentive for services. Thirty years later the inverse care law still prevails, implacably enforced by the system of no-system.

Concentration. When medicine was a cottage industry, the uninsured faced many barriers, but individual physicians could choose to provide pro bono care on a small scale, and, in the aggregate, the number of uninsured served this way was quite sizable. Now that we are well into medicine's new economic revolution, the pressure for profitability in many large systems of care is closing the doors on the uninsured and concentrating them in public facilities.

Fragmentation. With a shrinking public sector and a disinterested market, identifying sources for a comprehensive range of services has become considerably more difficult. For example, except for patients with acute psychosis or suicidal intent, obtaining timely mental health services is nearly impossible in many publicly funded health care settings.

Evasion. Despite legislation to prohibit patient "dumping," it still occurs. To survive, it has mutated into a less visible form. Private hospitals are no longer shipping indigent patients off to public EDs in a taxicab. Instead, they now offer perfunctory treatment, forego any diagnostic procedures, and discharge patients with instructions to "follow up tomorrow with your primary care physician." They might as well be advised to see their personal banker.

Degradation. The inverse care law is not invisible to the uninsured. The system of no-system exposes patients to a number of transactions for which the price they pay is their own dignity, such as being turned away when they cannot pay in advance for services, waiting interminable hours for care, and coping with clinicians and staff who show them little respect. In overwhelmed systems, the people served become the problem.

It would be easy for our patients to conclude that they are worth something only as potential research subjects. The bulletin boards of our office feature equal numbers of flyers encouraging us to refer subjects for various studies and offering regrets that due to cutbacks or increased patient load, certain clinics will no longer accept new patients.

Fixing HMOs Is Not the Answer

The public knows that health care in the United States is in a meltdown phase. And they know it from personal experience. Tinkering around the edges with HMO incremental strategies will not solve the fundamental problem. As long as health care is treated like a market commodity, the abuses that have become notorious will dominate public discourse. . . .

It's time to reintroduce the subject of universal health care in the richest country in the world. Just ask the average person.

Kit Costello, *San Diego Union-Tribune*, July 19, 1998.

Resignation. Working within such a system slowly erodes professional standards, as clinicians yield principles to realities. What is practiced is the art of the minimal.

Amplification. Healthy systems maintain stability through self-correction: threats to the system's integrity activate compensatory mechanisms that restore stability. In unhealthy systems, disturbances may trigger a response that creates an even larger disturbance: an amplification loop in which things go from bad to worse. An example is the loop enabled by employer-based health care when an employee becomes seriously ill and is fired, thus losing his health insurance, and his access to medical care. COBRA [Consolidated Omnibus Budget Reconciliation Act] medical care protection is a mirage for the working poor, with an annual cost per family of more than $7000. And those in most jeopardy for being fired because of sick time are at the lower end of the socioeconomic spectrum, thus creating a synergy between the greatest risk and the greatest consequences. A similar dysfunctional response occurs when, as the cost of health care rises, employers take steps to reduce their medical costs, one of which is hiring more temporary workers not covered by medical insurance. These workers are disproportionately from low-income groups and are thus less able than others in the population to cope with rising health care costs.

The most important example of how problems are amplified in the system of no-system is seen in the public health care infrastructure, which is being stretched thinner and thinner, essentially being pulled apart by increasing numbers of uninsured on one side and falling revenues on the other. A vicious circle ensues of falling revenues leading to cutbacks in levels of service, driving insured patients to other facilities, causing a further fall in revenues. Medicaid managed care has been successful in mainstreaming patients to community health care providers, but with an unintended consequence of choking off one of the main sources of income for public facilities.

Maladaptation. The system of no-system does not exist in a vacuum. It is embedded within the health care market and society at large. As those responsible for providing services within the system of no-system cope with these larger structures, maladaptations ensue. Some of the maladaptations result from attempting to maintain services modeled after the mainstream market without sufficient resources or personnel. Others arise when public institutions' strategies to survive in the market distort the decisions about what services should be pursued, leading to the paradox of high-tech citadels in Third World-like communities.

Time to Rescue the Uninsured

In 1996, the *Bulk Challenge*, a leaky freighter with 4000 Liberian civil war refugees aboard, sailed along the coast of West Africa for nine days seeking a port while neighboring countries, already overrun with refugees, refused to accept the ship. The vessel had one toilet and little food or water on board. There was an outbreak of dysentery and people began to die. At the time, I remember thinking that for a cost equivalent to one MRI, one could save hundreds of lives on that boat. We are now in an analogous situation with the uninsured in the United States. The boat is overcrowded and leaky, and people are suffering for want of services.

It is time to rescue the 39 million Americans who are forced to seek care within the system of no-system. If there is to be universal health care, we cannot keep having the same dialogues about the government vs. the market, equality vs. liberty, efficiency vs. bureaucracy. Stripped of all the ideology, the need and the suffering are there, now, plain for all to see. Stop by my waiting room sometime and I'll show you.

"Free universal healthcare is never free."

Universal Health Care Is Not the Best Solution for the Uninsured

L. Dean Forman

In the following viewpoint, L. Dean Forman contends that a universal health care program would not work at the state or national level. He argues that it is unrealistic to expect any health care system to provide comprehensive coverage for all Americans. Further, universal health care is expensive—much more expensive than managed care critics will admit. Forman insists that the best solution for U.S. health care problems will come from the combined efforts of government, employers, providers, and insurers. L. Dean Forman is president of the benefits brokerage firm Genovese, Forman, and Burford Financial and Insurance in Sacramento, California.

As you read, consider the following questions:

1. According to Forman, what is the biggest promise made by a universal health care program?
2. What is required if a universal system has an overall cap on spending, in the author's opinion?
3. What two elements make up medical care costs, according to the author?

California Governor Gray Davis signed a bill that requires the state to look at options to create a universal health insurance program in California. Some recent presidential candidates have also suggested government-sponsored healthcare.

Health insurers haven't left yet, because the report isn't due until 2003. But don't expect carriers to stay, if the experiences from other states are any indication. President [Bill] Clinton made this a campaign issue and failed, but some states continued with the holy grail of universal care. Here are the results:

Universal Health Care Did Not Work at the State Level

• New Jersey passed individual health insurance reform making it easier for the uninsured. The cost for a $500-deductible 80/20 plan—where the insurance company pays 80 percent and the insured pays 20 percent—ranges from $16,880 per year with Blue Cross to $85,200 annually with Manhattan National Life. The average current cost is $30,000 to $35,000 per year.

• Kentucky guaranteed all health insurance coverage to anyone regardless of health status. Result: Forty-five of the 47 insurers left the state. Now the state is scrambling to reform the reform.

• Tennessee said, "Let's put them all on Medicaid" (Medi-Cal in California). Result: The program consumes more than one-fourth of the state's budget after a promise that it would cost less than the state's Medicaid program would.

Why? The state of Tennessee said it has 114,000 uninsurable people. By contrast, California has 21,400 people in our high-risk pool. How is it a state with one-sixth the population has five times as many uninsurables? Could it be free government insurance?

Over the next few years, you're going to hear many cries for universal health insurance. Don't be deceived.

Universal illusion: There's no doubt that the present system for providing healthcare has flaws and needs to change. But we must proceed carefully.

The biggest promise made by a universal healthcare pro-

gram is to provide comprehensive health coverage for all—
no more uninsured anywhere. This is a powerful and appealing concept, but is it realistic? Compelling arguments
say it isn't.

A single-payer system controls medical costs primarily by
limiting the price it pays for medical services. This is essentially the premise of Medicaid and Medicare, which account
for roughly 42 percent of every dollar spent on medical care
nationally.

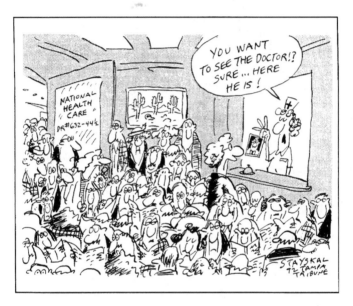

Stayskal. © 1992 by *Tampa Tribune*. Reprinted by permission of Tribune
Media Services.

These government programs work because they're national
and allow medical-care providers in each state to charge non-
government payers more to cover the underpayment from
Medicare and Medicaid.

If the United States set up a universal system, providers
could no longer shift costs from one payer to another. This
could substantially reduce provider income.

Also, most universal systems typically have an overall cap
on spending. This requires some form of rationing. If ra-

tioning in any form is unacceptable, a universal system won't be satisfactory.

Canada rations: For example, Canada pays most of its citizens' healthcare by using a set budget for hospitals and doctors' fees. Canadians are forbidden to seek government-provided services through private-sector healthcare. Here are the real tradeoffs.

According to the Vancouver-based Fraser Institute, 212,990 Canadians waited for a surgical procedure in 1998. This was 13 percent higher than 1997. The median wait for treatment was 13.3 weeks.

Provincial government budgets are set so low that demand outstrips supply. The result is that Canadians get to wait for their healthcare, if they can get it before they may die.

A Canadian friend had his mother diagnosed with cancer. Scheduling for follow-up tests would routinely take 30 days, followed by another 30 days for results. The doctor's response during the two-year ordeal, "You've lived a good life, you're 72 years old, we'll make you comfortable."

While he said they'd never state it directly, the underlying theme was, "We need to save our resources for the young."

Isn't that how you ration healthcare? Give it to the young who might benefit the most!

Universal Health Care Will Be Too Expensive

Who's going to pay? Let's consider the cost to taxpayers. Where will the money come from to fund the expansion of health coverage to Californians who don't have it now? And where will the money come from to pay for covering unemployeds and uninsureds from other states who may be drawn to California by our promise of coverage for all? Will there be enough money to give everyone unlimited healthcare access?

Free universal healthcare is never free. Taxes on gas, alcohol and cigarettes finance the bulk of the Canadian system. (In Canada, cigarettes are $5 a pack, gas costs $4.50 a gallon and cheap wine is $8 a bottle.)

Deceptive comparisons: Often, politicians base their criticism of the private healthcare system on their comparison between the cost of Medicare administration and their interpretation of the administrative costs of HMOs.

Per their statistics, the cost to administer Medicare is 2.3 cents per dollar of benefit. The HMO model's average administrative costs for profit-making HMOs is 13.6 cents, and 9.6 cents for nonprofit HMOs.

This comparison is wrong and grossly misleading. Consider:

• The 2.3 cents for Medicare administration represents only the cost of processing claims and the allocated budget expense of the Health Care Financing Administration, which administers Medicare. It doesn't include the cost of the large government bureaucracy that is involved in the Medicare program. In the private sector, both direct and indirect administrative costs are included in the administrative expense charge.

• The data do not include Blue Cross-Blue Shield administrative costs. Any study of insurer administrative expenses should include the largest health insurer in the nation.

• The data do not include any of the large self-funded plans administered by commercial carriers. This is typically the largest portion of most carriers' health business, and it is the least costly to administer per dollar of benefit.

In essence, studies selected a small part of the insurance industry's health insurance business for comparison—the part that costs most to administer.

• HMOs include marketing costs in their administrative expenses, and none is included in the Medicare expense figure.

• HMOs' expenses include taxes and fees; these aren't part of the Medicare expense figures either. A proper comparison of Medicare vs. HMO charges would exclude taxes and fees.

• HMOs include in their administrative charges the cost of their efforts to contain medical costs. Medicare does little or nothing to contain medical costs, opting instead to control prices paid to HMOs.

The most recent failure in this regard is the continuing pullout of HMOs in the Medicare risk marketplace. This was due to the unilateral decision by government to reduce payments to HMOs for Medicare patients.

Costs can still decline: HMOs can and will cut their administrative costs further. But I don't believe that reductions in such costs should be of the magnitude critics suggest of the private healthcare system. There aren't as many potential productivity improvements as they'd have us believe, nor is the public well served by providing the lowest level of service possible.

But there is value in having consultants/brokers involved. They help the public understand their options and coverage, and they help insureds interact effectively with the system.

Also, remember that medical-care costs are composed of essentially two elements—administrative costs and benefit costs. By all measures, the biggest piece is benefit cost.

We need to keep our focus on the entire animal, not just the wagging tail. We should not be afraid to spend expense dollars if it will save even more benefit dollars.

There's no "magic bullet." Rather, there's a series of things we must do together. Government, employers, providers and insurers can solve the many problems that affect healthcare if we work together with a common resolve.

It won't be easy, quick or perfect. Done right, however, it will be uniquely American, and better suited to our needs than anything off the shelf of another country.

"Tax credits should be a cornerstone for a renewed push to universal health coverage."

Tax Credits Should Be Used to Expand Health Insurance Coverage

Jeff Lemieux

In the following viewpoint taken from his testimony before the House Committee on Ways and Means, Jeff Lemieux argues that tax credits—health insurance subsidies to low-income workers—play a key role in the immediate expansion of health care coverage to the uninsured. In addition, tax credits can play an integral role in the eventual conversion to a system of universal, work-based coverage. The newly unemployed, he maintains, must maintain their coverage so that the number of uninsured Americans does not increase. All Americans, Lemieux insists, must have good health care choices at reasonable group rates with assistance given to those with low incomes. Jeff Lemieux is a senior economist at the Progressive Policy Institute.

As you read, consider the following questions:
1. According to the author, why have efforts to get universal health care coverage failed in the past?
2. What two characteristics must tax credits have to be effective at reducing the number of uninsured Americans, according to Lemieux?
3. What is the biggest flaw in the Bush administration's proposal for permanent tax credits, in Lemieux's opinion?

Jeff Lemieux, testimony before the House Committee on Ways and Means, U.S. House of Representatives, hearing on "Using Tax Credits to Expand Health Insurance Coverage," February 13, 2002.

The Progressive Policy Institute (PPI) has long argued that tax credits should be a cornerstone for a renewed push to universal health coverage. That is not to say that tax credits alone are enough to do the job—they are not. We will also need expanded safety net programs and greatly improved purchasing pools or other purchasing arrangements so that people can use their tax credits in an efficient, fair, and secure market. But tax credits are an important building block.

People sometimes roll their eyes when I talk to them about universal coverage. Haven't we tried that every decade for generations, and failed each time? I think past efforts to get universal coverage have failed mostly because they caused uncertainty about the fate of employer-based health coverage, which Americans value very highly.

However, I believe universal health coverage can be achieved this decade in a series of responsible, practical stages that enhance rather than threaten work-based health insurance.

The first step is to help the newly unemployed maintain their coverage. By preventing those with insurance from losing it when they lose their jobs, we can at least stop the number of uninsured from rising.

The second step is to actually reduce the number of uninsured by making certain that all Americans have good choices of health insurance at reasonable group rates, that they can exercise those choices in the most convenient and secure setting possible (usually their place of employment), and that financial assistance (based on tax credits) is provided to help those with low incomes.

To be effective at reducing the number of uninsured, lax credits must be both refundable—that is, fully paid even to those whose incomes are so low that no income tax liability is owed—and available "in advance," when people need the money to purchase their coverage.

Both the House-passed proposal for temporary tax credits for displaced workers and the Administration's proposed permanent tax credits for individual coverage pass the tests of refundability and payment in advance.

The temporary tax credits in the House-passed proposal for displaced workers also seem to me to pass the crucial test of not threatening employer-based coverage. However, I believe the Administration's proposal for permanent tax credits for individual health insurance could in fact disrupt employer-based coverage, and should not be enacted in its current form.

Temporary Tax Credits Should Be Increased

I have some suggestions to improve both proposals: . . . I encourage committee members to increase the temporary tax credits for displaced workers from 60 percent to 75 percent or more, to better ensure that few workers would lose health coverage and that employers' overall health costs would actually be reduced. Furthermore, we need to make sure that those temporary tax credits follow people when they get a new job, but are in the waiting period before they become eligible for coverage at the new job. Second, the Administration's proposal for permanent credits for individual health insurance should be expanded to include employment-based coverage, and should also be made available through payroll deduction at the workplace.

The biggest flaw in the [George W. Bush] Administration's proposal for permanent tax credits is that it doesn't allow people who get health coverage at work to receive tax credits, even if their incomes are very low. That is unfair, since low-income people who struggle to afford work-based coverage would get nothing. They would have an incentive to drop out of their employer's coverage or switch to other (often higher paying) jobs that don't offer coverage.

In general, businesses that don't offer employee benefits like health insurance can afford to grant higher wages instead.

Tax Credits Are a Path to Universal Coverage

Under the Administration's proposal, low-income workers would have a particularly strong incentive to take higher wages instead of employment-based health benefits, and then use the tax credit to purchase individual coverage. To save their employees the hassle of switching into no-benefit jobs to take advantage of the Administration's credits (and to retain valued employees), some small businesses would just

Over a Dozen Tax Credit Bills Have Been Introduced

There is considerable interest among policymakers in providing tax credits to individuals who do not participate in an employer's plan toward the purchase of their health care coverage. This would enable them to receive a tax benefit they do not currently receive but that workers who have employment-based coverage do receive. Recent research conducted by Mark Pauly and Bradley Herring of the University of Pennsylvania's Wharton School of Business found that a tax credit equal to 50 percent of premiums would reduce the number of uninsured by half.

In June 1999, House Majority Leader Richard Armey (R-TX) and Representative Pete Stark (D-CA)—the self-described "congressional odd couple"—agreed in an opinion editorial published in *The Washington Post* that uninsurance is the "biggest health problem facing the country." They also agreed on the root causes of uninsurance—a workforce that is "increasingly mobile and part time" and a perverse tax code that "discriminates against not only insurance purchased outside the workplace but also lower paid, part-time and small-business workers." They promoted the idea of refundable tax credits as a "bipartisan remedy."

Indeed, among Members of Congress, while there are some disagreements on the technicalities of tax credits, there is widespread bipartisan support for the concept itself. Over a dozen bills were introduced in the House and Senate during the 106th Congress to establish such tax credits. These bills had a combined total of 72 cosponsors from across the ideological spectrum. Moreover, both then-Governor George W. Bush and then-Vice President Al Gore included tax credits in their presidential campaign platforms.

Regardless of the technicalities, Congress should make the tax credits fully refundable, pre-payable, and available to all Americans.

James Frogue, *Heritage Foundation Backgrounder*, February 16, 2001.

stop offering coverage in the first place.

The better path toward universal coverage is to make mainstream group coverage affordable—through tax credits—and easily available at every workplace (whether or not the employer helps pay for coverage).

Even our friends at the Heritage Foundation, which has previously proposed radically individualized health insurance, are now publishing papers on how tax credits can be used and administered—at least as an option—through the workplace.

To sum up, the PPI strongly supports the effort to make refundable tax credits an integral part of a renewed drive toward universal health coverage. Tax credits shouldn't favor employer or individual health coverage. The current tax law favors employment-based coverage, especially for high-income people, but the Administration's proposal of permanent tax credits only for individual coverage is an overreaction, which strongly favors individual coverage for lower-income workers. The right policy would have a better balance. Tax credits should be available in both markets, so that both markets are strengthened.

"*The latest version of [health care tax credits]. . .represents bad tax policy, bad welfare policy, and bad health policy.*"

Tax Credits Should Not Be Used to Expand Health Insurance Coverage

Tom Miller

In the following viewpoint, Tom Miller insists that tax credits are just another name for income redistribution, and they will not help solve the problem of uninsured Americans. He maintains that giving health insurance subsidies to low-income workers through refundable tax credits will likely be financed by reducing current health coverage tax benefits for higher income workers. Miller argues further that tax credits reinforce the mistaken opinion that everyone is "entitled" to health insurance and that adequate medical care cannot be accessed without it. Tom Miller is the director of health policy studies for the Cato Institute.

As you read, consider the following questions:
1. In Miller's opinion, what are the politics of the health care tax credit issue?
2. What does the Republican health care tax credit strategy fail to provide, according to the author?
3. What does Miller suggest is the real reason that tax credits are not considered "welfare"?

This year's [2002] installment of Washington's chronically superficial health-care debate resumes. With the return of Congress, the "new" idea will be refundable health tax credits for displaced workers. But the latest version of this concept, passed in an economic stimulus bill in December 2001 by the Republican-controlled House, represents bad tax policy, bad welfare policy, and bad health policy. Standard operating procedure on Capitol Hill.

The politics of this health care issue are fairly simple. After the September 11, [2001,] terrorist attack [on America] pushed the economy into a deeper recession, both major political parties sought to express their compassion for workers who lost their jobs and found their health-insurance coverage in jeopardy. They also hoped to score some points that might advance their respective health-policy agendas.

Democrats opened with a legislative push to 1) expand government-run Medicaid assistance to displaced workers who lost access to employer-sponsored health plans and 2) provide even more lavish new subsidies to other laid-off wage earners who chose to continue their coverage under their past employer's plan (so-called COBRA [Continuation Omnibus Budget Reconciliation Act] continuation coverage). This two-step strategy first hoped to convince voters that only greater federal spending and federal control for health insurance coverage could keep the ranks of the uninsured from swelling further. Second, if neither politically controlled universal health coverage nor a greatly expanded Medicaid program could be achieved, at least the employer-sponsored health-insurance system could be propped up further to serve as a platform for new mandates, hidden cross subsidies, and future scapegoating. Employer group plans keep most workers locked up in a narrow range of insurance arrangements and deterred from wandering off our over-regulated "private/public" health insurance reservation. They serve as second-best host organisms for political parasites.

Republicans Proposed a Temporary Tax Credit

The not-even-too-clever-by-half response from congressional Republicans was to let voters know that they "cared" too, but in a manner that limited budgetary costs and headed off any direct expansion of the troubled Medicaid program. In December 2001, House Republicans and the George W. Bush administration placed their political bets on refundable tax credit assistance to many (but not all) displaced workers and their families. Eligible workers could obtain an advance income-tax credit (or an end-of-year credit) for 60% of their monthly premium payments for private health insurance.

At best, this proposal temporarily blocked an explicit expansion of Medicaid assistance to temporarily unemployed workers. It might open up some new private health insurance choices for them beyond the expensive COBRA coverage available from most of their former employers. Current COBRA benefits allow workers who leave jobs to retain group coverage for at least 18 months, but they must pay the full price for it without any tax benefits. Only about 20% of all eligible workers actually pick up this option. Employers complain that those who do exercise COBRA rights tend to run up larger insurance claims. Their costs exceed the maximum premiums allowed by more than 50%. Workers leaving jobs at companies that never offered health insurance or employed fewer than 20 people have no rights to any federal COBRA benefits at all.

But the Republican health care strategy misses the big picture for reform, while surrendering principles and just handing out more money.

It fails to provide new health care choices and tax parity to employed workers who don't participate, or do not want to remain, in their current employer's health plan. The Republican game plan begins and ends with targeted handouts, instead of broad, individual-empowerment reforms.

Even on the compassion front, only idle workers who are eligible to receive unemployment benefits would qualify for the Bush administration's refundable tax credits. In some states, that figure may be as low as one-third of all unemployed workers.

Government Tax Neutrality Is the Goal

If the real policy goal is neutrality for government tax treatment of health insurance, the solution is to exclude the cost of health insurance purchases from a worker's income that is subject to income and payroll taxes. Instead, Republicans have cobbled together an uneven policy mix: A tax exclusion (i.e., deductibility based on one's marginal tax rate) for the many employees of firms providing group insurance, and a tax credit for other purchasers of individual insurance policies that is fixed at a single rate (60%) that is higher than any taxpayer's marginal rate, but capped in total amount.

Tax Credits Are Risky

Tax credit proposals for the uninsured vary substantially in their details, and the details determine their ultimate impact. But the tax credit approach, absent substantial reforms of the individual market, holds grave risks for the future of the country's health care system. At worst, tax credit proposals could undermine the employer based health care system (ultimately destroying it), and drive up the ranks of the uninsured. Absent reforms of the individual market, individuals and families with significant pre-existing conditions could find that they do not have access to affordable, comprehensive coverage in the individual market. If coupled with so-called market reforms such as HealthMarts and Association Health Plans, the standard of benefit coverage could erode from today's relatively comprehensive employer-based plans to a standard of skimpy, bare bones coverage with high deductibles and limited protection. These are very real risks facing the health care system.

Consumers Union, March 11, 1999.

Even if the policy goal is to provide more of the current tax subsidy to lower-income workers, the real complaint should be with the progressive marginal tax rate structure of the current IRS [Internal Revenue Service] code. Until we move to a flat tax (the permanent solution), the value of any income tax deductions will always be greater for taxpayers in higher income brackets.

Most refundable tax-credit proposals (including those of the Bush administration and House Republicans) are designed to award tax "cuts" to individuals who pay little, or no, federal taxes. Yet it was less than a year ago [2001] that Republicans had to fight off political claims that the administration's tax-cut package was "unfair" because it provided most of its benefits to those who paid the largest share of federal income taxes. Duh. Endorsing a new round of income redistribution and federal spending via the tax code (in the name of "health care") is contradictory and counterproductive.

Another long-range danger of targeting health insurance subsidies to low-income workers through refundable tax credits is that they are likely to be financed, under budgetary pay-as-you-go norms, by reducing the current health insurance tax benefits available to higher income Americans. In effect, this means increasing the latter's marginal income-tax rates. Soak the rich, to subsidize the poor, for budget neutrality?

Health Insurance Is Not an Entitlement

Refundable tax credits endorse expansion of current taxpayer-financed "entitlements" to health insurance coverage. They reinforce the mistaken view that health insurance is a "merit" for everyone and that necessary access to health care cannot be adequately financed without even greater subsidies from taxpayers for insurance coverage. As the income-redistribution auction proceeds, additional political conditions on how these new tax subsidies for health insurance are to be spent will follow inevitably.

With federal welfare-reform law up for review and reauthorization, it's puzzling that many lawmakers— who salute the benefits gained from limiting the magnitude and duration of cash assistance to low-income beneficiaries on the welfare rolls—nevertheless appear poised to dole out a new round of permanent "welfare" checks to the working poor, hidden beneath a refundable health tax-credit label. Apparently, the stigma of welfare still can be applied to outright income support, but not other welfare payments routed through the tax code. Could it be because the primary beneficiaries of the latter really are health-care providers and health insurers looking to get paid more regularly by lower income customers?

Do greater tax subsidies to purchase more health insurance necessarily improve one's health? Interestingly enough, even though the self-employed receive less-generous tax advantages for health-insurance purchases than other workers and they are less likely than wage earners to be covered by health insurance, this relative lack of insurance doesn't affect their health. Craig Perry and Harvey Rosen concluded in a recent study for the National Bureau of Economic Research that "for virtually every subjective and objective measure of health status, the self-employed and wage earners are statistically indistinguishable from each other."

Passing Out Money Will Not Improve Health

In fact, simply passing out a new set of transfer payments via inefficient political filters won't substantially improve the health status of lower-income Americans. Recent research suggests that 1) improving quality of education that individuals receive, 2) cushioning vulnerable workers against sudden economic shocks, and 3) expanding individual control of one's health-care decisions will yield much greater returns. The real health policy reforms needed for dynamic change include:

- Broad tax parity for all health-insurance purchasers who pay taxes.
- Greater deregulation of health insurance alternatives.
- Expansion of defined contribution plans.
- Multiyear rollovers of flexible spending-account balances.
- Facilitation of voluntary group-purchasing arrangements outside the workplace.
- A surgical tummy tuck for the health safety net.

Instead, health-policy experts like Stuart Butler of the Heritage Foundation tell us that refundable tax credits are the ideal Left-Right compromise, because "liberals can vote for tax cuts and call them subsidies, while conservatives can vote for subsidies and call them tax cuts." A reality check indicates that someone's getting fooled in this political trade. Recent history suggests it's not the political patrons of the welfare state.

Before we point the tax-policy gun in a new direction, let's first make sure it's not aimed at our own feet.

"Our current employer-based coverage system is serving the nation well, and has the potential to be our most effective and expedient tool for substantially minimizing our national uninsured crisis."

An Employer-Based Solution Is the Best Answer for the Uninsured

Harry M.J. Kraemer Jr.

In the following viewpoint, Harry M.J. Kraemer Jr. argues that because over 80 percent of the uninsured population live in wage-earning households, the uninsured issue is really a workplace issue. The most effective solutions to the problem of the uninsured, he maintains, will be found within the existing employer-based health care system. He insists that refundable tax credits for the working poor, greater outreach programs targeting small businesses, and greater flexibility in the administration of public insurance programs must be part of the solution. Harry M.J. Kraemer Jr. is chairman of the Healthcare Leadership Council's Executive Task Force on the Uninsured.

As you read, consider the following questions:
1. According to Kraemer, what are the consequences of being uninsured?
2. What is the most significant barrier to insurance enrollment for low-income workers, in the author's opinion?

Harry M.J. Kraemer Jr., testimony before the Committee on Education and the Workforce, Subcommittee on Employer-Employee Relations, U.S. House of Representatives, hearing on "Expanding Access to Quality Health Care: Solutions for Uninsured Americans," July 9, 2002.

The members of the Healthcare Leadership Council (HLC) are committed to advocating a successful combination of solutions to solve the national [health care] crisis. We have both experience and ideas concerning reaching out to individuals and small businesses to begin reducing the number of uninsured Americans. And, through our grassroots initiatives, we are gaining additional insights in how to attack the educational and administrative barriers that stand in the way of broader health coverage for working families. I welcome and appreciate the opportunity to discuss the HLC's views and initiatives on this issue.

As I will discuss in my testimony, a large number of the uninsured in this country are workers in small businesses, and our efforts to address this problem must be focused accordingly. Our experience with the nation's public insurance programs—Medicaid, S-CHIP [State Children's Health Improvement Program] and the Qualified Medicare Beneficiaries' program—has taught us that simply making assistance available or providing financial subsidies does not, in itself, solve the problem. It is essential that funding efforts go hand in hand with complementary education and outreach efforts to maximize and ensure the effectiveness of any federal solutions for the uninsured.

Today, I want to discuss both the policy approaches that we believe will be most effective in helping working Americans gain greater access to health coverage, as well as the necessary outreach initiatives that must take place in order to achieve real progress on reducing the number of uninsured in our country.

The health care industry is, I am pleased to tell you, actively engaged in the mission of finding solutions to the problem of the uninsured. The Healthcare Leadership Council (HLC) is a coalition of chief executives of the nation's leading health care companies and institutions, representing all sectors of American health care. Our members are committed to advancing a market-based health care system that values innovation and that provides accessible, high-quality care for all Americans.

Last year [2001] the members of the HLC launched a national campaign called *Health Access America*. Our mission is to raise national awareness of the uninsured problem, and to advance solutions that will put health coverage within the reach of uninsured Americans. I speak for all of my fellow members and health industry CEOs in saying that we believe strongly that all persons should have access to today's modern medical miracles and life-enhancing technologies and treatments.

The health consequences experienced by those without health insurance are well documented. People without coverage tend to get sick more often because they do not receive the preventive and diagnostic care that so many of us take for granted. They miss more time on the job. They are absent from school more frequently and statistics recently released in an Institute of Medicine study tell us they will die too early.

This is a major social problem, and it is also an economic one. When a large percentage of our population is uninsured, our productivity suffers and our health providers are confronted with a tremendous economic strain caused by uncompensated care. Hospitals alone are absorbing over $19 billion per year in care provided to those who do not have adequate coverage.

It is critical to point out that there is no single answer, no one policy solution that will address the needs of more than 40 million uninsured Americans. Taking on this issue requires flexibility and a mix of targeted public and private solutions.

The HLC supports a three-pronged approach to reduce the number of uninsured Americans: (1) refundable tax incentives to encourage the purchase of insurance, including employer-offered coverage; (2) improvements to the current Medicaid program and S-CHIP, including improved outreach to enroll those currently eligible and the flexibility to use program dollars to expand private coverage; and (3) increased efforts to facilitate awareness of the importance and availability of health insurance, especially among the nation's small businesses.

We are focused intensely on this issue, and on making progress toward solutions. Under the auspices of our *Health Access America* campaign, we are spotlighting local and regional programs throughout the country that are developing successful, innovative approaches to help provide coverage. We are using our HLC Web page (www.hlc.org) to provide uninsured Americans with one-click access to information about coverage and safety net programs in their states. We are conducting research studies on the most effective ways to address this crisis. And we are talking to people who don't have health coverage, listening to their stories and sharing them with a wider, national audience to broaden awareness of the personal pain and the cost to society that will continue to be felt if we don't solve this problem.

I would like to share with you some of what we have learned, through our research, about the characteristics of the uninsured, and then discuss how we are using that knowledge. Of particular relevance to this hearing, I would like to discuss the very important objective of providing information to small businesses and working families on the value and accessibility of health insurance coverage. Finally, I would like to submit our views regarding two of the important components of expanding health coverage access—providing tax incentives to working Americans, and improving Medicaid and the State Children's Health Insurance Program (S-CHIP).

HLC has undertaken several research projects that are helping us to better understand the characteristics of the uninsured and potential solutions to the significant challenges before us. I would like to share a few of our most important observations:

Four out of every five uninsured persons are in families with at least one employed family member. This is critically important, because it alters long-held preconceptions about the uninsured and helps shape our policy approaches to address this problem. This is the dominant picture of the uninsured—hard-working people who are not offered or cannot afford health insurance. Of the 33 million uninsured in working families, 13 million are in families where an offer of insurance from an employer is turned down, usually because the family cannot afford it. Twenty million of the uninsured in working households are not offered employer insurance.

The cost of insurance, not surprisingly, is the most significant barrier to insurance enrollment for low-income workers and their dependents. This is in part because their share of premiums consumes a higher percentage of their income than is the case for workers with higher incomes. Also, workers in middle and upper-income brackets tend to work for employers who subsidize a larger portion of their health insurance premiums, whereas low-wage firms offer a smaller subsidy to their employees.

One Working Adult Provides Coverage

Despite an unprecedented term of growth in the nation's economy, the number of uninsured continues to climb. To help explain the conundrum of increasing rates of employment and prosperity along with decreasing rates of health coverage, HLC recently commissioned an analysis by The Moran Company of existing data on the uninsured. . . .

To further illustrate this, our study looked at how many individuals working in industries least likely to offer insurance actually receive insurance coverage through another family member. For instance, 77 percent of individuals working in the agriculture, forestry, and fisheries industry are not offered coverage by their employers. But 60 percent of these uncovered agriculture, forestry, and fisheries workers are covered by an insurance policy of another family member. Likewise, 53 percent of those in the sales industry sector are not offered insurance—but 60 percent of those uncovered workers in sales are covered elsewhere as well. That is to say that spouses and younger adults are able to accept jobs without an offer of insurance because they live within a family where one member works for an employer offering family coverage. As our report states, "the growing number of multi-earner families has a powerful mediating effect on the relationship between employment status and health insurance coverage." This data also helps to explain why a significant number of the uninsured are single adults.

Mary R. Grealy, testimony before the Senate Committee on Finance, March 13, 2001.

In all of our research, the single most important point that cannot be ignored is that the uninsured issue is a workplace issue, with millions of wage-earning households representing the lion's share of the uninsured population. It then stands to reason that our most effective solutions must be found within the existing private employer-based health care system. We believe strongly that the focus of our energies must be directed where it is needed most—toward the nation's small, Main Street businesses.

HLC's overarching belief is that consumers should have a variety of health coverage choices—in both the group and non-group markets. However, it cannot be overlooked that our current employer-based coverage system is serving the nation well, and has the potential to be our most effective and expedient tool for substantially minimizing our national uninsured crisis. Employers now insure over 64 percent—or about 177 million Americans. Not only are employers uniquely effective in pooling varied risks, but they also are a driving force in negotiating fair prices and quality improvement.

According to our research, more than 80 percent of the uninsured, or about 33 million uninsured individuals, are in families with at least one active worker. And most of these uninsured workers are employed by small businesses. At companies with fewer than 10 employees, about 33 percent of workers are uninsured; with 25 to 99 employees the figure is about 21 percent. In firms with 500 to 999 employees, only about 11 percent are uninsured.

As I mentioned previously, the primary barrier to health coverage for the uninsured is financing—for individuals and small businesses. However, there is growing evidence that the complexity of the small group insurance market and a basic lack of awareness about the value and cost of health insurance also act as significant barriers preventing small businesses from providing health insurance. . . .

While efforts to address the major financial barriers to health coverage must await legislative action, HLC and other private and public organizations can take action now to help break down the education and complexity barrier.

HLC has begun to develop regional initiatives targeted directly and specifically toward small businesses. Our goal is to help these businesses navigate the complexities of their local health insurance market in hopes that more, if not all, will purchase coverage.

For this Main Street Initiative, we are conducting an initial analysis of various small group markets. . . .

The information from each regional analysis will be used to design a set of outreach efforts for the region. These efforts will be aimed at increasing health insurance coverage among employees of small businesses. . . .

This is clearly an area in which the public and private sectors can work together to achieve considerable progress. Evidence has shown that greater access to information about health coverage can lead to more small employers providing that coverage and more working men and women electing to receive it. Those of us who are large employers can and must join with the public sector in making this education and outreach happen. . . .

Through our extensive grassroots program, the HLC is developing programs—in conjunction with community leaders—to provide local health briefings and forums, local media events, and awards presentations to model programs on the uninsured. . . .

While these regional efforts are vitally important, it is also critical that we establish sound national policies to make private health coverage more accessible for working families and to improve the effectiveness of the dollars currently devoted to federal programs like Medicaid and S-CHIP.

Targeted, Refundable Tax Incentives Will Help

Having established that the majority of the uninsured live within working, low-wage households, it is a logical conclusion that a pre-funded, refundable tax credit to lower income workers—for use toward group or individual insurance—could help to reduce the number of uninsured. Health coverage tax credits have the potential for providing consumers with a great amount of flexibility for choosing health coverage options that best suit their needs. They also can act as a stimulus to create new and wider coverage choices in the marketplace. . . .

The HLC believes tax credits should be refundable for persons with little or no tax liability, and they should be paid in advance so that individuals with limited or no savings can take advantage of them to pay monthly premiums before the end of the tax year. Risk-adjusting tax credits for those with chronic diseases and other health conditions, as well as facilitating the development of state high-risk pools toward which credits can be applied, can also help to ensure that the majority of the uninsured are served by this approach.

Refundable tax credits would be of tremendous value to low-income working families. The current tax exclusion for health insurance has less value for low-income workers than for their better-paid counterparts. For families with income levels between 200 to 300 percent of the federal poverty level ($35,000 to $53,000 for a family of four), the existing tax exclusion for employer-paid health insurance is worth only about $661. For families between 300 and 400 percent of poverty, the exclusion has a value of about $801.

While we are pleased to see proposals moving forward to use tax credits to address the needs of individuals who do not have an offer of employer insurance, it is our hope that these proposals will be expanded to include others in the workplace who face health coverage challenges. The HLC's strong advocacy for tax incentives to subsidize the purchase of employer-offered insurance stems from the compelling fact that over 80 percent of the uninsured are connected to the workforce. The combination of a refundable tax subsidy, the often lower cost of group health insurance and the natural outreach opportunities within an employment setting creates the most promising environment for increasing coverage for families and individuals.

Improving Medicaid and S-CHIP

Medicaid and S-CHIP have proven extremely valuable for providing health care to very low income populations, and must play a role in the package of solutions that will reduce America's uninsured population.

However, evidence suggests that we are reaching the limits of effectiveness in reducing the number of uninsured through these programs, as they currently function. Only about half of the individuals currently eligible for Medicaid and S-CHIP actually participate in the programs, suggesting that eligibility alone—without considerable investment to remove existing barriers to participation—does not and will not efficiently increase the number of people receiving coverage.

A number of reasons have been cited for low participation in these programs, including the fact that participation rates in means-tested public insurance programs decline as incomes rise. A large number of those electing not to participate are families with higher income levels who were offered public insurance upon the inception of S-CHIP. . . .

Any discussion of expanding S-CHIP or Medicaid eligibility must also take into consideration the deteriorating fiscal health of many of our states. Medicaid and S-CHIP account for the largest line item in most state budgets. And, unlike the federal government, virtually all of the states do not have the option of deficit spending, meaning that budget cuts will have to occur. The National Conference of State Legislatures' annual Health Priorities Survey for 2002 found that 28 states will consider cutting Medicaid benefit packages this year. Several governors have stated publicly that Medicaid spending is one of the greatest problems they face.

This challenging environment requires innovative approaches. For example, using S-CHIP funds to supplement employer premium contributions is a logical way to stretch scarce health care dollars. Virginia's FAMIS program, is one of the first programs in the nation to combine its S-CHIP funding with employer-offered coverage. This program is now enrolling thousands of uninsured children into their parents' health plans in the work place.

This idea should be examined closely by other states as well as the Federal government. Many eligible individuals in the higher income categories of Medicaid and S-CHIP, as well as income categories under consideration for Medicaid and S-CHIP expansions, are connected to the workforce through at least one family member. Therefore, solutions involving ways to supplement employer insurance may be highly effective in increasing coverage rates for these populations, providing coverage without the stigma of government dependence. There are steps that must be taken, though, to make this approach work better. There are administrative complexities within the Medicaid and S-CHIP programs that discourage states from opting to coordinate with employer health plans. HHS [Department of Health and Human Services] currently does not have the authority to eliminate all of these barriers. . . .

We firmly believe that the nation's uninsured problem is not an insolvable one. Through tax incentives, through improvements in our public programs and through intensive outreach and education to small businesses and working families, we can help more Americans achieve the key to longer, healthier lives that comes with having health coverage.

"Our plan would provide near-universal coverage among the non-Medicare population by making private plans more affordable."

Reforming Health Care Financing Is the Best Answer for the Uninsured

Sara J. Singer

In the following viewpoint, taken from her testimony before the House Committee on Ways and Means, Sara J. Singer argues that her new Insurance Exchange plan will achieve near-universal coverage by offering health insurance products that are a good value and accessible to all, with subsidies for those who cannot afford them. She insists that promoting competition among health plans by providing information about plan prices and quality will make them more affordable. A competitive market, she maintains, can manage expanded coverage at little cost. Sara J. Singer is executive director of the Center for Health Policy at Stanford University.

As you read, consider the following questions:
1. According to Singer, who would the U.S. Insurance Exchange serve?
2. What would be the function of the Insurance Exchange Commission, according to the author?
3. In Singer's opinion, what two features should any serious proposal for health care financing reform provide?

Sara J. Singer, testimony before the Subcommittee on Health of the House Committee on Ways and Means, U.S. House of Representatives, hearing on "The Nation's Insured," April 4, 2001.

Forty-three million Americans without health insurance is a serious and complex problem. . . .

To reduce the number of people who lack insurance requires both a health care system that delivers good value health insurance products given the dollars available and makes them accessible to all, as well as subsidies for individuals for whom the price of coverage is out of reach. Competitive models like the Federal Employees Health Benefits (FEHB) Program, the California Public Employees Retirement System (CalPERS), or Stanford University contribute to the first of these goals by offering multiple choices, structuring the competition among them, and providing incentives for individuals to select high-value plans (e.g., defined contributions). Though prominent and important examples, these purchasers represent a small minority of the health insurance market so by themselves they cannot be expected to transform the delivery system. Most employers offer one or few choices and pay more for more expensive health care plans thus weakening or eliminating incentives to choose economical health plans. Transforming health care delivery will require that providers actively seek ways to cut costs without harming quality. This, in turn, requires that a significant portion of their patients demand value.

My colleagues Alan Garber and Alain Enthoven and I, at Stanford University's Center for Health Policy, recently formulated a proposal to achieve near-universal health insurance by satisfying both requirements. We carried out this work as part of a project organized by the Economic and Social Research Institute and sponsored by the Robert Wood Johnson Foundation. In doing so, we sought to make a wide range of health insurance choices available to all Americans, to encourage consumers to seek high value coverage through improved competition and personal economic responsibility for choices, to increase support for care to those who remain without insurance, and to accomplish this without mandates on employers.

Affordability Is the Key to Coverage

Our plan would provide near-universal coverage among the non-Medicare population by making private plans more affordable. It would do so by using insurance exchanges to promote competition among plans. The exchanges would provide information about plan prices and plan quality, enabling consumers to make informed choices and obtain good-value health insurance. Our proposal includes the following key features:

• *Insurance exchanges* (public or private entities or employers) would offer individuals a choice of at least two health plans (one that provides some coverage for treatment by most providers, and a low-priced alternative) in every geographic region. Considerably more choices would be desirable, including point-of-service (POS) or preferred provider organization (PPO) products as well as closed-panel health maintenance organizations (HMOs) and newer alternatives such as defined-contribution "care groups." Non-employer exchanges would accept all individuals not eligible for Medicare and groups in their service area (guaranteed issue) at a flat premium rate (community rating), with adjustments only for covering additional people, such as a spouse or dependents. Exchanges would perform at least minimal risk adjustment (initial risk adjustment would be based on age) and/or rely on other mechanisms to limit the financial rewards to plans for engaging in practices that encourage risk selection, to preserve choice among plan types and create incentives for plans to enroll and care for high-cost patients. Exchanges would also participate in risk adjustment between insurance exchanges in a region or state. Exchanges would require quality measurement and would make available comparative information to help members make informed choices. Substantial incentives would encourage development of private exchanges. These include tying new subsidies to purchase of insurance coverage through an exchange, preemption from state insurance mandates (i.e., ERISA [Employee Retirement Income Security Act] protection), and protection from adverse selection.

• The *U.S. Insurance Exchange* (USIX), like the Federal Employees Health Benefits Program, would serve individuals and firms with fewer than 50 enrollees in areas in which private exchanges do not emerge.

• *Refundable tax credits* for health insurance valued at 70%

of the median cost plan for lower- and middle-income Americans (individuals with incomes up to $31,000/families up to $51,000, phased out for individuals with incomes between $31,000 and $41,000/for families with incomes between $51,000 and $61,000) who purchase insurance through an exchange. In contrast to families in higher tax brackets, today such households have limited financial incentives for purchasing private health insurance plans.

All Default Plans Will Be Federally Funded

• Individuals, eligible for tax credits, who do not enroll in a health plan, will be automatically enrolled in a *default plan* designated by the state to provide basic health care services. Default plans will be federally funded through performance-based grants initially equal to 50% of the tax credit. They will enable states to provide new financing for public hospitals, clinics, and other providers who meet standards of open access, as part of their default plan. States will receive incentive bonuses or reductions based on the extent to which they improve performance on a set of preventive care measures (e.g., childhood vaccinations, first-trimester pregnancy visits, hypertension control) and reduce the percentage of the population that remains uninsured. The goal is to ensure that every eligible individual is enrolled in a health plan.

• Other individuals would continue to exclude from taxable income their employer- or individually-paid health insurance, but a *phased-in cap* would limit this exclusion from taxable income for employer- or individually-paid health insurance benefits to encourage value-based purchasing. Individuals eligible for both the exclusion and the subsidy could choose which of the two tax benefits to use. The dollar value of the cap would be set high enough to represent a substantial subsidy, yet low enough to provide substantial new financing for expanding health insurance coverage and other purposes.

• A new, independent *Insurance Exchange Commission* (IEC) with narrow, specific powers, similar in function and structure to the Securities and Exchange Commission, would be created to distribute new subsidies and default plan payments, accredit insurance exchanges, conduct risk adjustment across insurance exchanges, and serve as a clearing-house for public information on the quality of health plans. This agency would have an appointment procedure and organization structure similar to that of the Securities and Exchange Commission, and would have a similar function—to encourage smooth information flow and functioning of insurance exchange markets.

Tax Credits Must Be Large

This proposal contains many similarities with the proposal offered by President George W. Bush as a candidate. The President's proposal, like ours, would use tax credits to expand coverage. The President's proposal differs from ours in that it offers smaller subsidies, targeted to lower-income individuals in employment groups without coverage. Unless they are larger, tax credits are unlikely to reduce substantially the number of uninsured due to low take-up rates and crowding out of employer-provided coverage. Even for individuals who receive tax subsidies, there may not be a viable market for these individuals to purchase coverage.

Uninsured Americans

The number of Americans without health insurance increased last year [2001] after two years of decline.

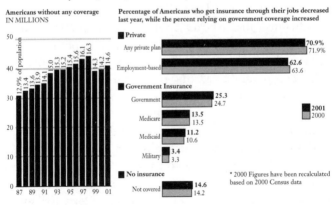

U.S. Census Bureau, 2001.

Adverse selection has made it nearly impossible to guarantee access to coverage and choice of plans to unaffiliated individuals in a system of voluntary health insurance. This is true despite attempts by the federal and state governments to ameliorate the problem through legislation providing for continuity of coverage for those who leave or change jobs and programs such as high-risk pools. The low level of subsidy proposed by President Bush would likely do little to improve the selection problem in an unstructured market.

The creation of a structured and competitive market through insurance exchanges can facilitate expanded coverage at little cost. Further, it can be an important part of any strategy to increase insurance coverage, whether subsidies are large or small. In addition, a system based on insurance exchanges would require little change if subsidies were expanded in the future to include more people.

The simplest approach to creating the benefits of an insurance exchange at the national level is the creation of one similar to the one available to federal employees. In our proposal, USIX would be a national exchange that would serve as an entry point for low-income, uninsured individuals, who would become eligible for new subsidies to purchase coverage. Like the FEHB Program, CalPERS, and Stanford University, USIX would offer competitive insurance choices. USIX could encourage development of high-quality coverage priced within reach of those eligible for subsidies. USIX would mitigate many of the market imperfections that plague the individual market (for example, through risk pooling, community rating, guaranteed issue, and competition). USIX could also determine limited benefit standards to provide reasonable comparability among plans and to prevent risk selection and segmentation. USIX would achieve economies of scale in brokering plans and would be capable of providing information about plan quality to individuals. Tax credits would promote higher-value health insurance options offered through USIX by exposing consumers to price differences.

A second feature of our original proposal worth consideration is automatic enrollment in default plans for subsidy-eligible individuals who do not enroll in a health plan. States would receive a payment initially equal to 50% of the new tax credits for these individuals and would apportion these funds to providers, such as public hospitals and clinics that they designate as default providers. States will receive bonuses or reductions based on performance. This mechanism would provide needed financing for safety net providers to care for those automatically enrolled in default plans as well as incentives for preventive care that should reduce hospital costs and expansion of coverage among subsidy-eligible individuals.

Any serious proposal for reform of health care financing should include elements of competition that encourage consumers to seek good value given the dollars available and subsidies for lower-income individuals. Our plan, like several similar plans, offers both and provides a path for further expansions in coverage in the future.

"I do not believe that our society can afford the continuing escalation of health care costs. But rather than denying people medical care, let us create options for the public."

Medical Savings Accounts Are the Best Answer for the Uninsured

J. Patrick Rooney, interviewed by Jerry Geisel

In the following viewpoint, taken from an interview conducted by *Business Insurance* editor-at-large Jerry Geisel, J. Patrick Rooney argues that because workplace-based Medical Savings Accounts (MSAs) offer an alternative to expensive managed care plans, they are a viable solution to the problem of uninsured Americans. MSAs, he maintains, provide low-premium, high-deductible health insurance to cover employees' catastrophic medical bills, and lets them use any other contribution their employer makes for health care as they choose. He insists that MSAs, available only to the self-employed or those working for businesses with 50 employees or less, offer employees greater control over their health care. Rooney is the owner of a company that sells MSAs in California.

As you read, consider the following questions:
1. According to Rooney, why will employees with MSAs use health care services more selectively?
2. Why did the tax law have to be changed for MSAs, in the author's opinion?
3. What formula does Rooney say employers should use to decide how much money to spend on MSAs?

Jerry Geisel, "J. Patrick Rooney: Promoting MSAs to Give Employees Greater Choice in Health Care," *Business Insurance*, November 3, 1997, pp. 94–96. Copyright © 1997 by Crain Communications Inc. Reprinted by permission.

Is managed care the only way to control health care costs and ensure quality? No, says J. Patrick Rooney.

Mr. Rooney, who led Golden Rule Insurance Company for nearly two decades before becoming chairman emeritus last year, has another idea: medical savings accounts linked to high-deductible health insurance policies.

Since the early 1990s, Mr. Rooney has been pushing MSAs, one of the few new ideas to emerge on Financing health care since the advent of managed health care.

The concept of MSAs is straightforward: set a very high deductible. Then, the employer contributes some of the premium savings to a special account. Employees can withdraw money from the account to pay uncovered health expenses or keep the funds for their own use.

With that financial incentive, employees are more likely to use health care services carefully, while still retaining the ability to choose their own health providers, Mr. Rooney said. With such a system, employees will be happier and more productive, he adds.

For Mr. Rooney, MSAs are more than a theoretical concept. Golden Rule, which was founded in Lawrenceville, Illinois, by Mr. Rooney's father and today has its major operations in Indianapolis, Indiana, adopted MSAs for its own employees in 1993. And the company lobbied Congress to gain tax-favored status for MSAs, which paid off in 1996 when Congress passed legislation giving MSAs established by small employers new tax breaks under a pilot program.

Mr. Rooney, 69, today has started a new insurance company. Medical Savings Insurance in Long Beach, California, which sells MSAs. He recently discussed MSAs and other health care issues with [Business Insurance magazine] editor-at-large Jerry Geisel.

Promoting MSAs Since 1990

Jerry Geisel: You have been one of the most ardent supporters of medical savings accounts. How and when did your interest in MSAs begin?

J. Patrick Rooney: I was in Washington and heard a speech at a program given by the National Federation of Independent Business Foundation. There was a professor there who discussed a rudimentary idea.

It didn't have a name. At that time it was not called medical savings accounts. But he said: "Why don't employers buy insurance for the big bills of employees and give them the savings, which could go into an account for employees and could accumulate?" You cut out the insurance company entirely on these small bills. That would give employees a financial interest—at least in the small bills—because if they spent more wisely there would be money that would accumulate in their own account.

When was that?

That was in November 1990. I had the advantage that I had resource people that could work on the idea. We went back and developed it in the spring of 1991.

Medical Savings Accounts Can Help Uninsured Americans

We need to radically improve access to health-care in this country. Recent estimates suggest that as many as 40 million Americans are without health insurance. To find a solution to this problem, our leaders must realize that a "one size fits all" mentality is no longer an option.

Medical savings accounts (MSA's) are one way to approach the problem of the uninsured. These programs, which were initiated in 1997, have provided a method to allow individuals to purchase a high deductible insurance policy, and allowing tax free contributions to a savings account to help cover the cost of that deductible.

Michael Burgess, www.burgessforcongress.com, 2000.

What was the reaction of the market when you unveiled it?

It wasn't unveiled at first to prospective customers. I went to Rep. Andy Jacobs (D-Ind.), with the idea. I said to him that the problem with this idea is that if people buy insurance, it is tax-deductible. The money they put into the savings account under tax law would have to be taxable income to the employees. I said to Representative Jacobs that we ought to change the tax code so that the decision would be neutral from a tax standpoint. He immediately said that is a wonderful idea. The first place we offered it to was employees of Golden Rule. I said if it is such a wonderful idea, why don't we offer it to ourselves. And we did. We took a lot of precautions to make sure no one felt strong-armed. We had a lower level management person hold meetings to explain the idea. Employees were each given pads in which they could personally calculate their medical care costs and whether or not it was going to be advantageous to them. We gave them a choice. We proposed to them giving them a catastrophic plan that would begin after $3,000. After that, it would pay at the rate of 100%. We would put $2,000 into the savings account. We explained to employees that there was a drawback. We told them that we would have to go to the payroll department and tell them we are putting this money into your account and they will withhold from your paycheck the taxes on the $2,000 we are putting in. More than 80% of employees chose to do it right off the bat. It is up to 93% today.

Happy with MSAs

How do you measure the performance of the plan compared with what you had before?

We don't have any good measure of the performance except in terms of employee satisfaction. There is no question that employee satisfaction is much higher. I never have had a situation before in my life that employees have stopped me and told me how much they liked our health plan. Since we put this in—at least in the beginning—I've had employees who stopped me in the hallway or elevator to tell me how much they liked it.

For employees, there are at least two obvious advantages. The medical savings plan provides first-dollar benefits. If you are an employee who doesn't manage your money well and you have a sick child you don't have to worry about a deductible. If you take your child to the doctor, you have first-dollar benefits. In addition, employees can use the account for other kinds of medical care that the insurance does not normally cover. For example, our employee plan never has covered dental and vision care. If you discover your daughter needs orthodontia, you can pay for it out of your medical savings plan. The employees like that very much. We have had several separate surveys of employees. Those surveys have shown high employee satisfaction connected with the fact that I can get my eyeglasses paid for and I can get my dental work paid for, and if there is money left over, it is my money. The underlying theory of an MSA is that I will have an incentive to use medical care services more carefully because I get the money in the account and because I have a big deductible.

But does the individual really have the knowledge and the clout to deal with providers to get the best deal?

Two answers to that. Yes. I believe they do. Secondly, there is a learning effect. Today, I being the consumer—I being illustrative only—don't have the knowledge or I am timid and don't want to ask ahead of time, the doctor might bark at me. There is a learning effect. You learn from your co-workers.

Some critics of MSAs say they are great for young, healthy people, but that the older, less well employees will—if there is a choice—stay in the traditional indemnity plan or the HMO. The next effect would be that the employer's health care costs really haven't changed very much.

It may. It doesn't have to. My argument is that an enlightened employer will want employees happy and satisfied with the health care plan. If employees are happier and more satisfied, that has utility to me as the employer. The first issue is, do the employees like it better? Incidentally, it may save money.

So, saving money is incidental? What is paramount is that employees have choice and can save money if they use services carefully?

Yes.

Smaller Firms Find MSAs Appealing

If MSAs are appealing to employees, why haven't more large employers established them?

My opinion is that the people making the decisions within the corporations believe that the employee is not capable of making the decisions. There is a lack of intellectual confidence in the employees. They think the way to control things is to create financial incentives so that the doctors that run the HMOs or whoever is answering the telephone will exercise better oversight of the employees. I'm positive of the ability of human beings to learn either immediately or to learn eventually.

It seems smaller firms are more receptive to MSAs. Why?

You have more of the entrepreneurial personality (at smaller firms). "Oh, I understand." That is kind of the classic response. Or, "It makes sense to me." I'm talking about a boss or owner, very likely someone who built the business.

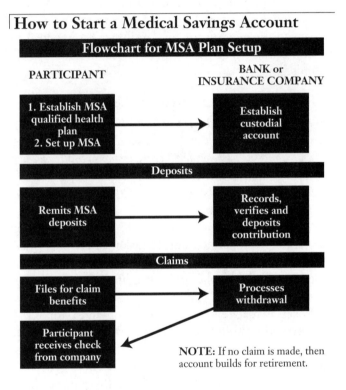

How to Start a Medical Savings Account

Flowchart for MSA Plan Setup

PARTICIPANT	BANK or INSURANCE COMPANY
1. Establish MSA qualified health plan 2. Set up MSA	Establish custodial account
Deposits	
Remits MSA deposits	Records, verifies and deposits contribution
Claims	
Files for claim benefits	Processes withdrawal
Participant receives check from company	**NOTE:** If no claim is made, then account builds for retirement.

Successful Farming, March 15, 1997.

Golden Rule was very aggressive, i.e., lobbying and advertising, to get Congress to change the tax law—and ultimately it has—albeit in a limited way, as it applies to MSAs. Why were you so passionate about this?

I think that is reflective of Pat Rooney's personality. I am a missionary. My fundamental statement on this subject is that we have to do something that is more rational to control health care costs. I do not believe that our society can afford the continuing escalation of health care costs. But rather than denying people medical care, let us create options for the public.

My company offers a PPO. When I go to a PPO doctor, the price is set and it usually is much lower than the doctor's normal charge. Doesn't that seem to be a more effective way to control costs rather than have individuals try to negotiate prices?

I would change the world more. I'm not sure it is the only effective way. I have asked what I would want for my family. I would want protection for my family for big medical bills. But I would want to throw the insurance company out of the small bills.

The Public Lacks Information About MSAs

In 1996, Congress gave MSAs tax-effective status, but limited the number of accounts that could be established to 750,000. After four years, Congress will decide whether or not to continue the program. Is that long enough or big enough to prove how well MSAs do or do not work? [On December 11, 2000, Congress extended the program until December 31, 2003.]

I don't think that had much to do with the decision. I think it was a political decision between the Democrats and the Republicans. But granted the current state of the public knowledge and the public understanding of medical savings accounts, it may well take a couple of years before the 750,000 cap is reached. Let me give you an example. I met with a very prominent Republican from Orange County, California. He is devoting his career to managing politics for the Republicans. He leaned back and said he was sorry that he had to admit this, but he said, "You are going to have to tell me what medical savings accounts are." Business writers ask me the same thing. The problem with medical savings accounts is that the public doesn't know about them or understand them. Indeed, Dr. Paul Ellwood [cofounder of the HMO concept] told me the same was true for HMOs in the beginning.

Do you see that 750,000 cap being lifted one day, and if so, why?

Sure. Any idea like this that gets this much conversation is going to happen. . . .

Are there some companies that shouldn't have MSAs?

I don't know of any reason why any firm should not have them. I would give it to employees as an option. I would not ram it down their throats.

MSAs Are a Rational Option for Health Care Financing

The program has to be designed very carefully. If the employer puts too much in the MSA, the employer can end up spending more than before. Isn't that so?

I'd suggest that the benchmark for the expenditure is the amount of money that now is being spent on the existing health plan. Some employers, when they go to the medical savings plan, cut back on the expenditure. They put in less money in the account than I would have them do. My opinion is that if you create increased employee satisfaction, that already is a big deal. Employers are not so benevolent that they would provide this if it wasn't a matter of employee satisfaction. There are employers who, when they go to the medical savings plan, cut back on the expenditure. I think that is a mistake. I would choose to put the same money into the medical savings plan and the high-deductible plan—the two would add up together to be the money that is already being spent. If I put more money in the savings account than I thought was really necessary, then I'd say, 'Oh, that is a gain in employee satisfaction.'

So, what should motivate the employer to set up MSAs?

It should be happier employees. I'll treat employees as adults. Let them make decisions for themselves. Out of this, Mr. Employer, the employees will know you treated them with dignity and they will have the opportunity to pay you back.

What do you see as the future of medical savings accounts?

They will be seen as a rational alternative. Rational, well-informed people will prefer to have this as an option. They will have a much more significant share of the market.

Periodical Bibliography

The following articles have been selected to supplement the diverse views presented in this chapter.

Meredith Alexander — "Stanford Health Policy Experts Offer New Health Insurance Proposal," *Stanford Report*, July 17, 2001.

Eric G. Anderson — "Lessons America Should Learn from a Land of 'Free' Health Care," *Managed Care*, January 1997.

Phil Benjamin — "Health vs. Wealth: The Struggle for National Health Service," *Political Affairs*, July 2002.

Sue A. Blevins — "Put Health Decisions Back Where They Belong," *Christian Science Monitor*, December 31, 1997.

Linda J. Blumberg — "Expanding Health Insurance Coverage: Are Tax Credits the Right Tack to Take?" *Urban Institute Online*, August 12, 1999. www.urban.org.

Bill Brubaker — "Co-Pay, or You Pay?" *The Washington Post National Weekly Edition*, August 5–11, 2002.

Christopher Byron — "A Cure for Health Costs: For a Limited Time Only, a Health Care Plan That Could Save You Plenty," *Esquire*, January 1997.

Richard F. Corlin — "The Time Is Right to Fix the Problem of the Uninsured," *American Medical News*, January 21, 2002.

Paul Ellwood — "A Cure for the Common Health Care System," *Imaging Economics*, August 2000.

James Frogue — "Top Ten Ways to Fix America's Health Insurance Market and Expand Coverage," *Heritage Foundation Backgrounder*, February 16, 2001.

Jon R. Gabel, Kelley Dhont, and Jeremy Pickreign — "Are Tax Credits Alone the Solution to Affordable Health Insurance?" Commonwealth Fund, May 2002. www.cmwf.org.

Medicine and Health — "Giving Credit Where It's Due: Tax Credits and the Uninsured," April 22, 2002.

Robert B. Reich — "The Case (Once Again) for Universal Health Insurance," *American Prospect*, April 23, 2001.

Sharon Smith and Paul D'Amato — "Health Care in the U.S.: A Sick System," *Socialist Worker*, November 21, 1997.

Leo M. Stevenson — "MSAs vs. Universal Insurance," *OB GYN News*, November 15, 1999.

CHAPTER 4

How Should the United States Reform Its Health Care System?

Chapter Preface

Bipolar disorder, schizophrenia, depression, obsessive-compulsive disorder (OCD), attention-deficit disorder (ADD), post-traumatic stress disorder . . . once these were terms heard only in a medical school lecture hall or on the psychiatric floor of a major hospital. Now they are dinner table conversation, the topics of television features, and first-person stories in the Sunday paper. The human mind—sick and well—became the focus of scientific research, media exploitation, and political attention when Congress declared the final decade of the twentieth century the Decade of the Brain. In 1996, with popular and political interest fixed on mental health, Senators Peter Domenici and Paul Wellstone decided the time was right to introduce their Mental Health Parity Act (MHPA). This act established parity between the annual and lifetime benefits that employees suffering from mental illness received and the benefits received for medical and surgical care. Although the act did not require employers to offer mental health benefits, it did require parity if such benefits existed.

Both Domenici and Wellstone had close family members suffering from mental illness. They were familiar with the emotional pain it could cause as well as the financial hardship that resulted from uninsured mental health treatment. After intense debate, Congress passed the Mental Health Parity Act of 1996, and it became effective on January 1, 1998. Domenici and Wellstone were not surprised to learn that the insurance inequities outlined in their bill were echoed by the 1999 Surgeon General's Report on Mental Health in America. According to the report, "There is an enormous disparity in insurance coverage for mental disorders in contrast to other illnesses."

The surgeon general's report also noted that at any given time, about 20 percent of the U.S. population is affected by mental disorders. Depression alone affects about 19 million adults. Even though over 90 percent of suicides can be linked to untreated mental illness, less than one-third of adults suffering from a diagnosable mental disorder, and an even smaller number of children, receive any treatment at all. Without the Mental Health Parity Act of 1996 to ensure equitable insurance benefits, most people would not be able to afford the help they need. Improved drug treatments and more effective therapies for mental illness, the result of scientific research prompted by the Decade of the Brain, would therefore be unavailable to those who need them most. Russ Newman of the American Psychological Association Practice Organization contends that "health care coverage in this country needs to catch up with what people increasingly understand . . . the mind and body are linked inextricably, and the perpetuation of discrimination against mental health in benefit design makes no financial sense and no common sense."

The Mental Health Parity Act of 1996 was written with a "sunset clause" and expired on September 30, 2001. President George W. Bush signed an appropriations bill early in January 2002 that contained a provision extending it until the end of that year when new debates on an expanded mental health parity bill would take place. The struggle for a solution to mental health parity was just one of the challenges that emerged during the Decade of the Brain that did not end with the start of the new millennium. Issues of mental health cost and accessibility continue to plague the American health care system. It is no coincidence that the High School National Debate topic for the 2002/2003 school year was "Resolved: That the United States federal government should substantially increase public health services for mental health."

The debate about mental health policy will rage on in Congress as well as in high school auditoriums. It is just one of the areas where government initiatives might improve the U.S. health care system. Authors in the following chapter examine several others, from those allowing patients to sue their HMOs to those allowing doctors to join unions. Their arguments test old laws and new theories as they struggle to make the health care system better, more responsive, and more accessible to all.

"There are too many lives to be saved and too much illness to be avoided to reject the medical ID."

Medical IDs Would Improve the Health Care System

David Orentlicher

In the following viewpoint, David Orentlicher argues that a "unique health identifier," or medical ID, would save many lives and improve the overall health of most Americans. He maintains that complete computerization of each individual's health records would ensure that data from different places could be brought together quickly and accurately when needed. Orentlicher contends that strict privacy safeguards required to protect confidentiality could be put in place without difficulty; it is easier to limit access to computer files than to paper records. Orentlicher teaches at the Indiana University schools of law and medicine at Indianapolis.

As you read, consider the following questions:

1. What act called for the creation of a "unique health identifier," according to the author?
2. In Orentlicher's opinion, how would medical IDs help researchers?
3. Who should have access to an individual's medical information, according to the author?

The argument for a "unique health identifier" is simple and powerful: It will save many lives and it will improve the health of most Americans.

Congress called for a unique health identifier, or medical ID, in 1996 when it passed the Kennedy-Kassebaum Health Insurance Portability and Accountability Act. As Congress recognized, doctors can provide optimal medical care only with good information about diseases and treatments and full knowledge about their patients. However, medical data are scattered across millions of hospitals, laboratories and doctors' offices, and they are often in charts that are buried, misplaced or lost. Many patients are poorly treated and research is slowed because vital information is inaccessible,

If we assign medical IDs to everyone and move their health-care information from file drawers to computers, then physicians, researchers and public-health officials will be able to find the data they need to prevent, diagnose and treat disease. Computerization will ensure that medical data are preserved in a usable form. Medical IDs will ensure that data in different places can be brought together.

Consider just a few of the benefits of medical IDs and computerized health records. Your physicians can give you the highest-quality medical care. Imagine, for example, that you are on vacation in another state, 2,000 miles from home, when you pass out and are taken to an emergency room. The doctors in the emergency room need to know which medications you are taking, whether you have a history of heart disease, diabetes or other illness and whether you have any drug allergies. Without such information, the physicians might make the wrong diagnosis or dispense inappropriate treatment, causing serious harm or even death. Currently, there is no easy way for the doctors to obtain the information they need. They would not know which hospitals or clinics to call, and they may not have much time to figure it out. If you had a medical ID and your medical records were computerized, however, the emergency room's physicians could access your records quickly through the hospital's computer.

Medical IDs and computerized medical records will improve the safety of the drugs on which you rely. Suppose you are taking a new anti-inflammatory medication that has dramatically eased your severe arthritic pain. However, because the drug was tested on only a few thousand patients, there may be serious side effects too rare to have been detected. In addition, since the drug was studied for only 12 months, there may be other serious side effects that take more than a year to show up. We won't know about these problems until the drug is in wide and prolonged use, and doctors make the connection between the drug and the side effects. In the meantime, you and other patients might be greatly harmed.

A Unique Health Identifier Could Provide Greater Privacy than Current Practices

In the midst of the differing opinions over what unique identifier might be acceptable and whether it is necessary, it is easy to forget the implications of current practices. Because identifiers differ across organizations, most health care records and transactions contain more elements of identifying information than might be necessary if a single unique identifier were used. Typically, health care records contain a patient's name, gender, address, phone number, birth date, SSN, health insurance number, employer, and relationships to other family members. A combination of several of these data items is often necessary to ensure a correct match between the records and a particular individual. In effect, a medical record or transaction bearing merely a person's name and address may make the information "open" to anyone who deliberately or accidentally comes in contact with it. Ironically, this use of personal information for matching people and records generates little controversy, despite the lack of security standards and privacy protections in place today. . . .

In addition, some believe that protection of health information from inadvertent or unauthorized disclosure would become easier with a unique individual identifier that is used for health care, but not for other purposes. . . .

From this perspective, an identifier that could replace other items of identifying information and that would be used only in health care might yield greater privacy protection than alternatives that do not share these properties.

U.S. Department of Health and Human Services, "Unique Health Identifier for Individuals: A White Paper," July 2, 1998.

It took five years and tens of millions of prescriptions before doctors realized that giving fenfluramine and phentermine—more commonly known as "fen-phen"—for weight loss could cause serious damage to heart valves. Only then were the two diet drugs withdrawn from the market. With medical IDs and computerized records, pharmaceutical companies could monitor the effects of their drugs much more easily and detect unexpected problems much more quickly. Indeed, with better monitoring, the companies also would detect unexpected benefits of their drugs much more quickly. Importantly, the companies could obtain the information they need anonymously. They could be given data about patients who take their drugs without knowing where the data came from.

Medical IDs and computerized records will improve health-care coverage. Assume, for example, that your employer offers a choice among three health-maintenance organizations, or HMOs. You have talked with friends who belong to the different HMOs, but you still don't have a very good sense of how they compare in quality, and your employer has provided you with information only about the differences in cost and coverage. If we had medical IDs and computerized records, it would be much easier for an independent watchdog group to collect anonymous medical data and provide critical information about the three HMOs: How long you need to wait to see a specialist; how well the HMO's patients do after heart surgery; how early the HMO's physicians diagnose their patients' cancers; and how many of the members leave the HMO each year because they are dissatisfied with the care.

Faster, Cheaper Research Is Another Benefit

There will be other important benefits from adopting medical IDs and computerizing medical records. By making it possible to retrieve complete medical data about patients, the medical ID and the computerized records would allow researchers to study diseases and treatments more quickly and more cheaply, thereby speeding up the development of cures. Better access to medical data would also improve the ability of public-health departments to do their work. They could detect new epidemics more promptly, and they could design more effective ways to prevent the spread of infectious diseases such as AIDS and tuberculosis. As with most other uses of medical information, research and public-health efforts could rely on anonymous data.

Of course, along with the substantial benefits of medical IDs and computerized records, there are real risks to individual privacy and patient trust. If medical information is more accessible to physicians, researchers and public-health departments, it also is more accessible to computer hackers, nosy hospital employees and law-enforcement officials. Patients may be less willing to disclose personal information to their physicians for fear that it will fall into the hands of others.

These are important concerns, but they are not reason enough to reject a medical ID. Without the ID, we avoid risks to privacy, but we also lose the many and considerable gains for the lives and health of Americans. It would be like throwing out the baby with the bath water. We would be better off by adopting medical IDs and also adopting strict safeguards to protect privacy.

Medical IDs Would Enhance Privacy

In fact, there is reason to believe that medical privacy would be protected better with medical IDs than without them. Under our current health-care system, confidentiality of medical information is porous. More than 15 years ago the ethicist Mark Siegler found that some 75 people had legitimate access to a patient's hospital record. Today, an individual's medical information routinely passes among physicians, health and life insurers, drug companies and employers. Yet, legal protection of medical confidentiality is weak. Federal law provides clearer protection of your video-rental records than of your medical records.

Because of the threat to medical privacy from medical IDs, the possibility of their creation has spurred members of Congress to become serious about the need for privacy protection and to propose real safeguards for medical information. We can expect an implementation of the medical ID to be accompanied by rigorous federal privacy legislation. Indeed, when Congress mandated the ID in 1996, it also called for national privacy protection through either federal legislation or federal regulations.

Opponents of the medical ID argue that the government cannot be trusted with personal medical information. However, nonprofit organizations rather than the government can store the newly computerized medical data.

In addition, even if the government could tap into the computerized records, opponents exaggerate the risks. For decades, the government has had access to the medical data of tens of millions of Americans: current and former soldiers who are treated in the military's or the Veterans Administration's clinics and hospitals; elderly and indigent persons whose health-care bills are paid by Medicare or Medicaid; and patients who participate in medical research at the National Institutes of Health. The government has acted responsibly in protecting the confidentiality of the medical information it already holds.

Strict Safeguards Are Required

The real question is not whether we should create medical IDs but which safeguards are needed to protect the confidentiality of medical information. There are several critical ways to preserve patient privacy. First, as almost everyone agrees, we should not use Social Security numbers as the medical ID. Social Security numbers are used as identifiers by too many private businesses to ensure sufficient protection.

Access to medical information must be strictly limited to those who have a legitimate need for the information. Then, when access is granted, it must be granted to only the relevant parts of the patient's medical record, if a health insurer is concerned about reimbursement for a patient's shoulder surgery, the insurer would not have access to information about the patient's breast cancer.

In fact, when medical records are computerized, it is much easier to limit access to specific parts of the medical record. When people peruse a paper record, they inadvertently may come across all kinds of information. On the other hand, when data are computerized, they can be given higher or lower levels of security. For example, a patient's psychiatric history could be highly restricted so that very few people would have access to it, while information about the patient's ear aches could be more accessible.

Information should be released in anonymous form for most uses. A treating physician needs to link data to a particular person, but researchers, public-health officials and drug companies do not need to know the names (or the IDs) of the patients from whom their data come. Finally, as required by the health-insurance portability act, there should be stiff penalties, including heavy fines and incarceration, for unauthorized intrusions into a patient's records. Such violations of privacy should be easy to detect since intruders leave unique computer "fingerprints."

There are too many lives to be saved and too much illness to be avoided to reject the medical ID. Rather, we must ensure that it is used in a way that protects both health and privacy.

*"With fully computerized records stored in a
central bank, the opportunities for . . . abuse
would almost certainly multiply—and so
would the actual incidence, particularly
without sufficiently strict privacy."*

Medical IDs Would Not Improve the Health Care System

Maggie Scarf

In the following viewpoint, Maggie Scarf contends that the
"Unique health identifier," or medical ID, is a dangerous
threat to personal privacy. Centralized storage of patients'
computerized health records would leave them vulnerable to
the most casual record browser and make doctor-patient
confidentiality impossible, she maintains. Moreover, Scarf
argues, if everyone's health information becomes part of a
national data pool for research purposes, the concept of informed consent—an individual's right to decide whether or
not to participate in research—will be destroyed. Scarf is a
contributing editor for *The New Republic.*

As you read, consider the following questions:

1. According to Scarf, which provision of the Kennedy-
   Kassebaum health care law worried some people?
2. What did over one-third of the Fortune 500 companies
   admit to using in making job-related decisions,
   according to the author?
3. In Scarf's opinion, who stands to benefit financially from
   the creation of "unique health identifiers"?

[In July 1993], when the public suddenly became aware of a controversial provision of the 1996 Kennedy-Kassebaum health care law, the reaction was swift and indignant. Buried deep within the otherwise innocuous bill, the proposal called for the creation of a permanent electronic health recorder—or "unique health identifier," as it would be known—for every American. Each person's record would have a complete medical history, and all of the records would be stored together in a central electronic vault with access controlled by the government. According to its proponents, this wonderfully efficient method of medical record-keeping would not only help doctors make better decisions—it would open vast new possibilities for research and cost-cutting.

The plan was quickly denounced by those who worried that we might be racing headlong into an Orwellian nightmare [where citizens will have no privacy at all]. Fine, the government would control access to the files. But according to what criteria? Within days, Vice President Al Gore announced a moratorium on the development of the unique health identifier until such time as strong patient-privacy legislation was securely in place. Then Congress, not to be outdone, put real teeth in the recommendation by cutting off all resources for the implementation of the unique health identifier until the close of the fiscal year.

The uproar ended there, but the story didn't. Indeed, under the original terms of the Kennedy-Kassebaum law, if Congress doesn't pass a patient-privacy protection bill by August 21, [1999, former] Health and Human Services Secretary Donna Shalala must draw up a list of regulations on her own, potentially clearing the way for a return of the identifier.[1] And, although nobody is quite sure what patient protections Shalala has in mind, a look back at a tentative, 90-page proposal she submitted to Congress in September 1997 provides a less than comforting impression.

Although Shalala asserted that there exists an "age-old right to privacy" and called for some important protections, she also argued in favor of allowing law enforcement officials

---

1. Congress did not pass a patient-privacy protection bill by the deadline. However, a moratorium was placed on the identifier, saying that no federal funds could be used to implement the plan until Congress approved its specific details.

or, under certain circumstances, "official[s] of the U.S. Intelligence Community" easier access to individual records. In addition, she provided a long list of others who could gain access to health records—from next of kin to researchers to insurance company clerks—whenever they cited "health care and payment purposes." In other words, Shalala's guidelines would allow for all sorts of access to these confidential records by all sorts of people—and, unless Congress or the administration intervenes, those guidelines will likely shape the final privacy regulations. "We are really at a crossroads," says Richard K. Harding, M.D., a child psychiatrist and privacy advocate who serves on the citizen's committee advising Shalala. "Centuries of medical practice, founded upon such strong ethical principles as patient-physician confidentiality and informed patient consent, are in the process of being tossed out the window, but no one seems to realize it or even be paying any attention."

There are several rationales for allowing such wide access to personal information. One argument is that rapid transmission of information would enable health care providers to look quickly at a patient's complete medical history in an emergency and discover, say, a past disease or medical allergy that might help identify an otherwise ambiguous affliction. In addition, it would enable better—and faster—research of health care in the aggregate. "We could look at cost-effectiveness carefully—analyze who has access to the various health services and what kind of services they are," says Georgetown University law professor Larry Gostin, an expert in the field of public health and a proponent of the unique health identifier. "We could also look at hospitals in terms of how well they are functioning, and we could assess the efficacy of various kinds of medical procedures. There would be many clinical benefits, both for patients and for research." Proponents of the unique health identifier also assert that it will help prevent fraud and abuse, since the government would have an easier time tracking claims records, just as it would produce efficiency gains for insurance companies—electronic billing is less costly than paper billing. (Not surprisingly, some of the identifier's loudest advocates on Shalala's advisory board represent the insurance, data collection, software, and research industries.)

These are all worthy goals—but they'd be purchased at a steep price. Consider, for example, the identifier's repercussions for psychiatry. Who, after all, would confide his or her deepest fears, embarrassments, fantasies, and dilemmas to a clinician knowing that these most intimate secrets would be shipped off electronically to Washington, where any of a variety of people could access them for any of a variety of purposes? There are also aspects of physical treatment that a patient might understandably prefer to keep confidential—such as being tested for a sexually transmitted disease, having an abortion or a mastectomy, or suffering from a terminal illness. Medical technology is discovering all sorts of ways to identify who's at risk for genetically transmitted diseases. In the wrong hands, though, that information could cost somebody his or her insurance coverage—or even a job.

Of course, medical privacy has been under attack for a while, thanks to the increasing computerization of patient records and the growth of managed care, which relies on detailed information to make decisions about treatment and coverage. Once a patient has signed a standard insurance release in order to get benefits, his health records become available to electronic file clerks, case managers, and insurance administrators, not to mention the physicians and nursing staff working in that patient's HMO or employer-owned insurance plan. Frequently, employers are also privy to medical histories: according to a 1996 University of Illinois survey, more than one-third of the Fortune 500 corporations that responded admitted to having used their employees' medical files in the course of making job-related decisions, such as promotions. (Moreover, it's possible that many respondents had done so but didn't admit it, making the true number even higher.)

This is why many psychotherapy patients, alerted to the current privacy threat, already elect to go outside their health plans and pay for treatment out of their own pockets. These individuals don't want the things they say in therapy to be used against them in the future; often, they don't even want it known that they've sought psychological treatment at all. But, if a unique health identifier is put into play, there won't even be a secure place "outside the system." As Robert Pyles, president of the American Psychoanalytic Association, puts it, a national identifier would function as a kind of "national tattoo." He explains: "Many people have the comfortable notion that if you're not a celebrity—someone like Bill Clinton, whose intimate life became a national spectacle—your personal information won't ever get you into much trouble. But it's the ordinary citizens who need to realize that there are very serious ways in which access to their medical information can impact upon their lives and their careers."

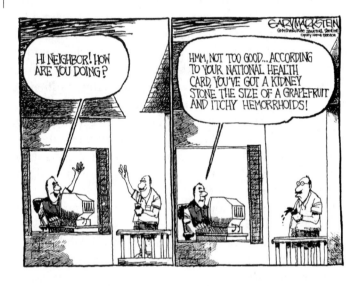

Markstein. © 1998 by *Milwaukee Journal Sentinel*. Reprinted by permission of Copley News Service.

If, for example, someone with a health problem applies for a job—and if his potential employer can see his medical records—he may not stand a chance against a healthy applicant, who'd be less likely to drive up the firm's insurance premiums. Or, if a person with a very substantial salary is applying for a home loan and someone has figured out how to access her medical history, she may be refused that mortgage because she has suffered from depression or gone through a bout of cancer. Such fears may sound outlandish, but anecdotes of compromised privacy are not hard to find even now, without the unique health identifier. In one incident described in the November 23, 1995, *New England Journal of Medicine*, a Maryland banker who was sitting on a state health commission used data about his bank's debtors to figure out which ones were suffering from cancer—and then called in their outstanding loans.

An even more infamous episode, reported on the front page of the October 8, 1992, *New York Post*, occurred when the medical records of congressional candidate Nydia Velazquez were faxed anonymously to a number of media outlets three weeks after she had won the Democratic primary in her district in 1992. The records showed that Velazquez had, one year earlier, voluntarily admitted herself to a Manhattan hospital after a serious suicide attempt. As the congresswoman (she went on to win the election and now represents New York's twelfth congressional district) later testified in a Senate hearing on high-tech privacy issues: "For the press, it was a big story. For me, it was a humiliating experience over which I had no control. . . . Very few people knew about my situation, and I [had] made the decision of not sharing it with my family. . . . My father and mother, eighty years old, they did not understand. They still do not understand."

Velazquez is simply one of the more high-profile victims of what Brandeis University medical ethicist Beverly Woodward has termed "record browsing." As Woodward has noted, "Documented cases of browsing by insiders in large computer networks indicate that the behavior is not uncommon . . . and that it may be carried out for such diverse reasons as curiosity (e.g., about friends, neighbors, relatives, or celebrities), perversity (e.g., sexual interests), anger (e.g., on the part of an employee who is about to be or has recently been dismissed), or a desire for financial or political gain." With fully computerized records stored in a central bank, the opportunities for such abuse would almost certainly multiply—and so would the actual incidence, particularly without sufficiently strict privacy protection.

Surely the most compelling argument for the use of identifiers is the potential gain for research. If it would really save thousands of lives down the road, surrendering a bit of privacy doesn't seem like such a sacrifice. But the true irony here is that the reams of information a unique health identifier would generate might not even be all that reliable in the long run. That's because, as privacy advocate Paul Appelbaum, M.D., says, "if we were to implement unique identifiers, you'd soon find everyone engaged in subverting the system in every way they could." For example, doctors uncomfortable in their role as government informers might conspire with patients by reporting as little accurate medical information as possible, and patients, once they'd wised up to the privacy threat, might withhold important data from physicians.

The real problem with the research argument, though, is that it stands in direct opposition to the most fundamental principle of research involving human subjects: informed consent. If all of our health information becomes part of a vast national database—freely available for medical studies and for business-related cost-cutting analyses—none of us would have a shred of choice when it came to our willingness to participate, or our wish not to participate, in such research. We would all, in effect, become "human subjects."

Alas, such lofty abstract arguments are not likely to persuade the other groups lobbying for the creation of identifiers—large computer, data bank, and telecommunications corporations. These wealthy, powerful companies see vast profit potential in the collection, organization, and sale of health care data. According to a May 10, [1999,] article in the *Los Angeles Times*, drug companies and hospitals already spend up to $15 billion a year on technology to acquire and exchange medical information about us, such as our blood pressure and the psychiatric medications we may be using.

Huge profits can be realized by easing legal access to our health data; and, as Charles Welch, M.D., the chairman of the task force that developed the Massachusetts Medical Society's patient-privacy and confidentiality policy, recently said, "There is a long gravy train forming around our medical records." Eager investors, including database companies, insurers, and the managed care industry, stand to reap millions—while the rest of us stand to lose not only our insurance, our jobs, and our money, but our privacy and our personal dignity as well.

*"Immunizing HMOs against liability
claims simply conceals the social costs borne
by patients when under-investment in
quality of care brings suffering, pain,
disability and sometimes death."*

Patients Should Be Allowed to Sue Their Health Plans

William B. Schwartz

In the following viewpoint, William B. Schwartz argues that the main purpose of a medical malpractice suit is to deter future negligent behavior rather than compensate the current victim. He maintains, therefore, that patients should be allowed to sue their HMOs. Only when HMOs are forced to decide that it is less expensive to change their practices than to pay damages when a judgment goes against them will they become accountable for their decisions, Schwartz contends. William B. Schwartz is a professor of medicine at the University of Southern California.

As your read, consider the following questions:
1. In Schwartz's opinion, what is the most useful criterion for judging medical negligence?
2. What act prevented HMOs from facing the possibility of a malpractice suit, according to the author?
3. According to Schwartz, what do opponents argue will happen if managed care organizations are opened to malpractice suits?

William B. Schwartz, "The Correct Rx to Target Malpractice," *Los Angeles Times*, March 15, 2000, p. B-7. Copyright © 2000 by Los Angeles Times Syndicate. Reproduced by permission.

Whether patients will be allowed to sue HMOs for malpractice finally will be resolved by a congressional conference committee pitting a nominally supportive House against a recalcitrant Senate. Despite the House vote eliminating the immunity of health maintenance organizations from claims of negligence, the chances of new legislation emerging soon are small because the speaker has stacked the committee with members unalterably opposed to any change.

The clarity of the debate is being obscured because neither side appears to understand the fundamental purpose of the malpractice system. They each start with the erroneous assumption that compensating victims of medical negligence is the main goal of malpractice law. In fact, the real purpose is to deter future negligent behavior by putting health care providers on notice that negligent care can result in severe economic penalties.

Negligence Must Be Proven

Yet what constitutes negligence? The distinguished Judge Learned Hand many years ago laid out the most useful and widely accepted criterion, stating that "negligence occurs whenever it would cost less to prevent a mishap than pay for the damage predicted to result from it."

As an example, let us say that there is a sudden failure of a light on the stairway of a store. In the following moment or two, the darkness causes a patron to lose her footing and fall, breaking an arm. No jury is likely to find negligence on the part of the owner because it would not be reasonable to station an individual on every stairway to provide instantaneous correction of lighting problems; the cost would far exceed the anticipated costs of any injury, calculated as the probability of the injury occurring multiplied by the cost of the injury. If, however, someone takes a fall after the light is allowed to remain unrepaired for half an hour or more, the situation is different because the cost of checking on the light at relatively long intervals is low. Preventing the accident would have been far less costly than the cost of the injury to the shopper. Under these circumstances, a jury would be expected to find for the plaintiff.

Yet this sensible act of balancing costs of prevention against the costs of injury is exactly what HMOs can avoid. Because of an unexpected consequence of the Employee Retirement Income Security Act, or ERISA, HMOs do not face the possibility of malpractice suits no matter how egregious their behavior. Health care providers thus have no motivation to offset their desire to maximize profits. Without risk of penalty, they are spared the need to invest in reasonable measures to prevent harmful outcomes.

Not Every Injury Requires Compensation

Immunizing HMOs against liability claims simply conceals the social costs borne by patients when under-investment in quality of care brings suffering, pain, disability and sometimes death. Barring lawsuits may help keep premiums low, but it simply shifts the burden to the patient and eliminates a highly desirable deterrent to improper refusal of HMOs to pay for care.

Cost Is Not the Real Issue

The HMO advocates say that patient lawsuits will increase costs. . . . First, even if lawsuits raise costs, that is immaterial when they are necessary to rectify improper conduct. Second, it is not clear that responsibility and accountability raise costs. The opposite may be true. Accountability and responsibility will require a more efficient and well-managed operation that should lower costs. Third, even if costs to the HMO are raised, they are likely to be more than offset by lower costs to the patients. When HMOs refuse proper treatment for patients, that simply raises patients' out-of-pocket expenses and the costs to society in unnecessary death and injury.

Herb Denenberg, *The Denenberg Report*, July 2, 2001.

As the light bulb example demonstrates, someone who is injured is not automatically entitled to compensation even though everything about the injury is identical to that of another person who does merit compensation. Nor does this formulation of malpractice law mandate that all injuries be prevented. If the cost of prevention is greater than the anticipated damages, avoiding the injury is simply not economically feasible. Over-investment in safety is not justified because it misuses society's resources. With most HMOs enjoying virtual immunity from patient lawsuits, the key problem is under-investment, not over-investment.

Opponents of opening managed care organizations to malpractice suits argue that HMOs will become victims of a flood of capricious lawsuits that will drive up premiums. Such an outcome is highly improbable. Lawyers who take on malpractice cases usually do so on a contingency basis, meaning that they don't get paid unless they win. Why would they take on lawsuits that are not winnable and impose heavy, non-reimbursable expenses on themselves?

On the other hand, patients and lawyers who do bring valid claims will be acting as unwitting but valuable agents of a broader social good. The prospect of financial reward for plaintiffs and their lawyers provides the incentive for them to play their part in making HMOs accountable for their health care decisions.

If the ERISA protection against patient claims is repealed and HMOs react rationally to the threat of lawsuits, they will be forced to use the Learned Hand calculus in making appropriate investments in patient-care quality. That's good news for all HMO patients, not just those who win in the courtroom. [As of October 2002, ERISA was not repealed and no legislation had been passed allowing patients to sue their HMOs.]

"*The HMO that calls 99.9% of the cases correctly could be bankrupted by decisions deemed incorrect after the fact in 0.1% of the cases.*"

Patients Should Not Be Allowed to Sue Their Health Plans

Richard A. Epstein

In the following viewpoint, Richard A. Epstein contends that allowing patients to sue their HMOs would be disastrous. Costs would skyrocket, he maintains, because patients would sue their HMOs whenever care was denied. Moreover, the cost of lawsuits and damages would force some HMOs into bankruptcy while others would have to raise premiums, pricing many employers out of the market and leaving their employees without health care, he argues. Richard A. Epstein is a professor at the University of Chicago Law School.

As you read, consider the following questions:
1. According to Epstein, no business should remain in operation if its own revenues cannot cover what?
2. What information did elaborate HMO databases provide, according to the author?
3. According to the author, modern studies are virtually unanimous in concluding what about HMOs?

One of the major initiatives on today's policy screen is to expose health-maintenance organizations to tort liability for patients' bad medical outcomes. Last month [September 1999] California enacted legislation expanding HMO tort liability. In Washington, Reps. Charlie Norwood (R., Ga.) and John Dingell (D., Mich.) are leading the charge to remove the federal statutory barriers to tort suits against employer health plans that improperly deny benefits to its members.

At the same time, the state courts have joined the chase on two theories. The narrower theory, which tracks the Norwood-Dingell bill, allows the patient to hold the HMO responsible for its own dereliction, typically its refusal to authorize some needed treatment. The more ambitious theory, just embraced in Illinois, holds the HMO vicariously liable for the physician's negligence, even if the HMO is guilty of no negligence of its own. Two arguments buttress this position. First, stringent HMO controls make physicians de facto employees of the plan, and not mere "independent contractors." Alternatively, the HMO holds itself out to its customers as being responsible for physician care by announcing, for example, that it will take care of "all your health-care needs" by supplying "comprehensive high-quality service."

Unsound General Rules for HMOs

The philosophy driving expanded liability is easy to discern. Brushing aside the prospect of increased cost, the Illinois court noted: "Market forces alone are insufficient to cure the deleterious effects of managed care in the health care industry." The court added that HMOs are subject to the same rules as everyone else. Part right, and part wrong. Right, because HMOs are not "special" organizations, governed by their own set of rules. Wrong, because Congress and the courts hold HMOs to unsound general rules.

Tough tort rules of liability make sense for protecting strangers from business misdeeds. The firm that pollutes the air or runs down an innocent pedestrian must be made to internalize the costs that it imposes on others by assuming liability, thereby preventing the firm from receiving forced subsidies from the people it injures. No business should remain in operation if its own revenues cannot cover the costs it inflicts on outsiders. In this context, principles of vicarious liability and negligence strengthen the market system by counteracting the implicit liability subsidy.

Patients, however, are not strangers to the HMO. They have an opportunity, either alone or in groups, to enter into contracts that specify in advance the level of services provided and the fees to be charged for those services. Where's the market failure when both parties to the transaction have the incentive to seek the right level of care for the right price? Using employers and other third-party agents stops clever HMOs from duping gullible employees who overlook the fine print in their contracts.

In this setting, each extra dollar of damage payments and litigation expenses at the back end requires fresh funding at the front end. To cover their higher costs, HMOs must raise fees and lose market share as employers pull out from plans that are now priced for more than they're worth. Alternatively, the HMOs get hit by price controls, at which point they exit the field unless bankruptcy gets them first. It's no accident that the number of uninsured moves up hand in hand with each new legal mandate.

Old Arrangement Promoted Excesses

Physicians, who chafe under HMO practice restrictions, may cheer the HMOs' pending demise. But their patients should be suspicious about this new celebration of physician autonomy and the familiar claims of inferior medical service. The HMO is no cute marketing trick. It responds to serious structural flaws in the old deals whereby third-party insurers signed blank checks for whatever services conscientious physicians ordered. That cozy arrangement induced excessive, and often unnecessary, amounts of medical care: "better safe than sorry" sounds great when someone else pays the bill. The HMO helped address both problems. Its increased level of service review cut out some of the excesses. Furthermore, elaborate HMO databases often provided solid information as to which treatments worked, and which did not.

The right question to ask is not whether HMOs misfire. It is whether they perform as well as the next-best alternative. Viewed in the round, the modern studies are virtually unanimous that HMOs, on average, provide care equal to that under the older fee-for-service system, and at a lower price. Surveys also indicate that most members, most of the time, are satisfied with the care they receive.

Liberalizing Lawsuits Will Increase Costs

Estimates are that liberalizing lawsuits against HMOs will cause premiums to increase by up to 12%. With HMOs struggling at net margins of 2% to 4%, something has to give. Remember, 10% of a trillion-dollar industry is $100 billion. It is no wonder that trial lawyers look at this opportunity so lustfully.

Robert R. Larsen, *Postgraduate Medicine*, February 1999.

The demonization of the HMO in today's folk culture doesn't depend on detailed knowledge of success or failure in any given case. The problem lies in the law of large numbers. Any system that enrolls tens of millions of members is sure to produce some injustices and outrages. These stories quickly make it to the front pages and the legislative hearings. The success stories are forgotten as the pressure builds for reform that in fixing outliers imperils the system as a whole.

Markets, by contrast, respond to the predicament that people find themselves in before the fact. It asks them to choose coverage and price levels before they know their individual health needs. But after tragedy occurs, no rationing of health care is satisfactory. Desperate patients demand pricey specialists, expensive procedures and experimental treatments.

Checking Function

HMOs were born because their members want both effective care and low prices—which requires HMOs to act both as providers who give care and as gate-keepers who can deny excessive care. If direct tort liability were cost-justified, then HMOs would voluntarily adopt it. But imposing unwanted tort liability on the HMO impairs its ability to discharge that critical, if unpleasant checking function. Individual physicians and practice groups can be counted on to defend themselves from charges of medical malpractice by saying that the

HMO made us do it. The HMO that calls 99.9% of the cases correctly could be bankrupted by decisions deemed incorrect after the fact in 0.1% of the cases.

When the dust settles, the supporters of the new tort initiatives will conclude that failed markets must be replaced by direct government provision of comprehensive health care, uncontaminated by the crude profit motive. They will neglect to mention that these "market failures" were driven by a network of government regulations of which tort liability is only the most conspicuous. Yet when government health care is besieged by liability, the next wave of reforms will immunize the government programs from tort liability.

Our object lesson: market failures, so-called, lead to government regulation, while failed government regulation leads to, well, more government regulation. An outraged American public that gets what it wants may get what it deserves.

*"Our only hope for protecting people from
the greed and abuses of managed care may
be the unionization of doctors on behalf of
their patients."*

Physicians Should Be Allowed to Unionize

Glenn Flores

In the following viewpoint, Glenn Flores argues that the advent of managed care has made unions necessary for doctors. Faced with denial-of-care decisions, he contends, doctors working within the managed care system need the power of a union to be effective advocates for their patients. Unionizing, he maintains, will give physicians the collective strength they need to wrest medical decision-making power from managed care providers and allow physicians to do what is best for their patients. Glenn Flores is a pediatrician at Boston Medical Center and an assistant professor at the Boston University School of Medicine.

As you read, consider the following questions:
1. According to Flores, what aspect of their managed care plan worries 55 percent of patients?
2. In the author's opinion, what could happen to doctors who do not meet their productivity requirements?
3. What is the average salary of a managed care executive, according to the author?

Glenn Flores, "Doctors' Unions Will Protect Patients Against Abuses," *The Progressive Media Project*, June 1999. Copyright © 1999 by Glenn Flores. Reproduced by permission of The Progressive, 409 East Main Street, Madison, WI 53703, www.progressive.org.

L ike many in my profession, I chose to be a doctor so that
I could help people. I love the richness of life as a physician: preventing disease, curing illnesses, alleviating suffering and, most of all, helping fellow human beings in their
times of greatest need.

My vision of the ideal practice of medicine never included
membership in a union—until recently. A doctors' union
may be the only way to protect a patient's rights and ensure
quality health care for all.

The juggernaut of managed care necessitates such a dras-
tic step. Its very existence requires the maximization of profits for executives and shareholders at the expense of patients
and their physicians.

The goals of managed care are ostensibly to reduce costs
and eliminate wasteful spending. The sad reality is that managed care's blatant profiteering endangers the health of
many Americans, particularly the most disenfranchised—the
poor, the uninsured, the chronically ill, and minorities.

Denial of Care Can Cause Injury or Death

In a recent national survey, most Americans said that managed
care has reduced the quality of care for people who are sick
and decreased the amount of time that doctors spend with patients. An impressive 55 percent said that they are at least
somewhat worried that if they become ill, their managed-care
plan would be more concerned about saving money than
about what's the best medical treatment for them.

The list of managed-care abuses is long. Denial of needed
medical visits and procedures is the cornerstone of the cost-
containment strategy that managed care euphemistically
calls "utilization review." Serious injuries, permanent disabilities and even deaths have been caused by such denial-of-
care decisions. These decisions reveal the unfortunate "profits over patients" agenda that all too often characterizes
managed care. Linda Peeno, a former claims reviewer for
several HMOs, recently testified before the House Commerce Committee that she had denied a necessary operation
to save a man's heart. That denial caused his death. She was
not punished, she said. Instead, she was rewarded by the
HMO. As she put it, "Not only did I demonstrate I could do

what was expected of me, I exemplified the 'good' company doctor: I saved a half million dollars!"

Managed care's treatment of physicians also demonstrates that the dollar is usually the bottom line.

HMOs often have productivity requirements, such as seeing a minimum of eight patients per hour (an average of 7 minutes per patient). Bonuses greet the doctor who meets or exceeds these requirements, and salary deductions or dismissal may await those falling short.

Strict Rules Inhibit HMO Physicians

To join an HMO, physicians may have to sign "gag rules," prohibiting them from informing patients of treatments that might be most beneficial, but are considered too costly by the company.

"Medical red-lining" is a process by which a managed-care plan can rid itself of "unprofitable" doctors and their patients. For example, a physician caring for many minority or poor people is more likely to encounter a greater severity and prevalence of disease. Dealing with more illness means more treatment and more hospitalizations. An easy way for an HMO to reduce costs is to drop both the physician and his or her patients from its health plan.

Professional Membership in Unions Is Growing

Why the remarkable union growth among white-collar professions? Unions are reacting to efforts by companies and public agencies to subject professionals to the disrespectful treatment accorded blue-collar workers. All professionals want a voice in the workplace and opportunities to use their special skills without heavy-handed interference from bureaucrats. Increasingly, they are deciding that unions can give them some measure of protection against workplace insecurity.

Harry Kelber, *Inside the AFL-CIO*, April 10, 2001.

Frustration with managed care has led to efforts by physicians to unionize. The American Medical Association just voted to form a union for doctors who are salaried employees. About 40,000 physicians, or 6 percent of American doctors, already belong to unions. In response, health-insurance spokesmen are asserting that unions are only about boosting doctors' incomes, which will raise health-insurance premiums.

Managed-Care Executives Are Well Paid

The irony is that managed-care executives are some of the most well-paid in the world. HMO executives average $2 million per year in compensation, according to Families USA, a health-advocacy group. In 1997, the 25 highest paid executives in 15 of the largest for-profit HMOs made more than $128 million in annual compensation, an average of $5.1 million per executive.

The 25 executives with the largest unexercised stock-option packages in 1997 had stock options valued at $290.4 million, an average per executive of $12.6 million. These exorbitant annual executive compensations cost health-plan enrollees anywhere from $ 1.51 to $40.30 annually. In contrast, providing consumers with the right to independent appeal of health-service denials would cost between 4 cents and 84 cents per HMO enrollee per year.

Every day in my inner-city pediatric practice, I see children and parents who have no choice but to confront homelessness, violence, hunger and poverty. William McGuire, the CEO of United HealthCare Corporation, had a stock-option package valued at $61 million in 1997. I would love to see McGuire sit down with one of my families and explain why it is reasonable for him to earn tens of millions of dollars in one year, while they can be denied basic medical care and health insurance. Until that meeting happens, our only hope for protecting people from the greed and abuses of managed care may be the unionization of doctors on behalf of their patients.

"Putting patients first won't exactly dominate the agenda of any union of practicing physicians."

Physicians Should Not Be Allowed to Unionize

Joshua M. Sharfstein

In the following viewpoint Joshua M. Sharfstein argues that doctors only want to unionize so that they can bargain with HMOs for higher fees. Sharfstein insists that patients will be caught in the middle as physicians and insurers negotiate union contracts. Ultimately, he maintains, patients will pay the price in increased costs and diminished quality of care. Joshua M. Sharfstein is a fellow in general pediatrics at Boston Medical Center.

As you read, consider the following questions:

1. According to Sharfstein, which physicians' organization is in favor of unionization?
2. What happened when physicians collectively controlled the supply of medical services, in the author's opinion?
3. What does Sharfstein argue is the fundamental problem with the health care system?

Joshua M. Sharfstein, "White Coats, Blue Collars," *The New Republic*, August 2, 1999. Copyright © 1999 by The New Republic, Inc. Reproduced by permission.

It wasn't particularly surprising that the American Medical Association [AMA], in announcing its plans to organize the nation's physicians into a union, depicted the decision as one aimed at helping patients. "Our objective here is to give America's physicians the leverage they now lack to guarantee that patient care is not compromised or neglected for the sake of profits," declared Dr. Randolph D. Smoak Jr., chairman of the AMA board of trustees.

What was surprising, however, was that so many people expressed hope about the AMA's claim. The *New York Times*, for instance, editorialized in favor of the AMA's decision, noting that "for consumers, unionization may be a positive force if doctors use collective bargaining to negotiate for improved patient services rather than merely for higher physician pay." The state of Texas is even counting on it. [In July 1999], Governor George W. Bush signed a law that relaxes antitrust rules to allow groups of independent doctors to bargain collectively. Bush boasted that his state now "provides a check and balance to make sure that HMOs are not able to unfairly use their market power to dictate the quality of patient care."

Unfortunately, though, the track records of the AMA and physician monopolies suggest that putting patients first won't exactly dominate the agenda of any union of practicing physicians. The AMA, after all, is the same organization that fought for years against limiting the out-of-pocket charges doctors can bill Medicare beneficiaries. The AMA has also been willing to favor pro-tobacco legislators with its political contributions—even as it has singled out smoking as a public health threat—in cases where those legislators also support the financial interests of physicians.

Top Dollar, Not Top Care

As for physician monopolies, in the few places where physicians have collectively controlled the supply of medical services, they've focused more on winning top dollar for themselves than on top care for patients. For instance, when orthopedic surgeons in Delaware collectively boycotted the state's Blue Cross/Blue Shield program in 1998, the Justice Department alleges, the driving force was opposition to fee cuts—even thougn the insurer's new fees were still higher than those paid in nearby Philadelphia. Similarly, in Tampa Bay, 29 general and vascular surgeons formed a corporation to negotiate with managed care companies; the most tangible result of the negotiations was the $430,000 in extra pay they earned the physicians in 1997. "The participants in that scheme did not take any collective action that improved quality of care," Assistant Attorney General Joel Klein recently noted while voicing his opposition to antitrust relief for physicians before the House Judiciary Committee.

Even allowing that some new professional ethic or strict legislative arrangement might limit the ability of physicians' unions to negotiate prices, the conflict inherent in a labor market for physician services will threaten to undermine any potential benefit to patients. Perhaps the most telling example of what physicians' unions might mean in practice comes from a recent dispute between managed care giant Aetna and doctors in Louisville, Kentucky.

Aetna vs. Louisville Doctors

The trouble started in 1996, when Aetna began to require physicians who accept any one of its plans to accept all of them; Aetna's long-term goal is for employers to be able to switch among its plans without requiring employees to change physicians.

Normally, Aetna's significant market share would allow it to get away with this sort of thing and essentially dictate contract terms to individual physicians and practices. But, in Louisville, where 1,800 physicians have banded together to form an association called The Physicians, Inc. (TPI), Aetna met some stiff resistance.

[In] March [1999], TPI gave 120 days' notice that it would not renew its Aetna contract, saying that the proposed "all products" clause forced physicians to accept insurance plans that they were not prepared for and to agree to future plans not yet defined. In large part, the dispute was about control, but it also had potential implications for the quality of patient care. Forcing reluctant doctors to receive a fixed amount of money for just a few HMO patients creates a huge incentive to reduce the care provided them—or to provide such bad care that costly patients leave altogether.

Although TPI isn't a union, and its members are allowed to make their own deals with Aetna, as many as 1,000 Louisville physicians—backed by the local medical society and the AMA—prepared to drop their Aetna patients. It wasn't until June, after State Insurance Commissioner George Nichols III used the threat of an investigation to push Aetna to the bargaining table, that the impasse was temporarily resolved. TPI physicians had offered to see Aetna patients until employer contracts expired; under pressure, Aetna agreed to pay them until then or until March 31, 2000.

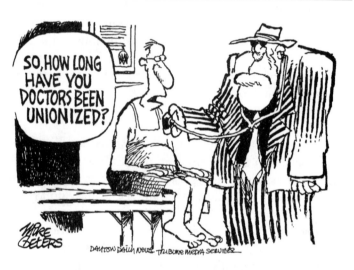

Seters. © 2000 by King Features Syndicate. Reprinted by permission.

From the market's perspective, the TPI/Aetna dispute has been a clear success. Aetna, acting in its own interest, attempted to force a contract provision on doctors. But TPI, acting in the physicians' interest (with some potential collateral benefit to patients), refused to agree to the ultimatum. Since neither side exerted monopoly power, both could walk away and plan to make other arrangements. That's how a balanced labor market should work.

From the bedside, however, the Louisville conflict has been a disaster. Thousands of area patients still face the loss of clinicians whom they trust with their health; that means that, sooner or later, some patients will have trouble finding and visiting new doctors. Compelling evidence exists that patients who do not have regular physicians have more trouble finding care in times of illness; in one recent study, having a regular physician better predicted access to care than did insurance status. About the only remedy offered to Aetna customers in Louisville comes from Nichols, who now advises them to follow some "consumer tips"—including asking their present doctors questions such as "What other insurance do you accept?" and "Does your office expect problems with any of these insurance companies that might cause you not to accept their insurance during the next twelve months?" There's nothing like asking whether you're about to be abandoned to start off the doctor-patient relationship on the right foot.

No doubt, many Americans are suffering from overzealous cost containment by insurance companies. But that doesn't mean we should suffer even more from disruptive conflicts between physicians' unions and insurers. The fundamental problem with our health care system is that it already relies too heavily on market forces—namely, insurance companies striving to increase their profits—to make reasonable decisions about the public good. Introducing yet another quasi-industrial mechanism—in the form of doctors able to use collective bargaining to increase their compensation—will be a particularly inefficient and unfair form of quality control. In the end, unionization may be the right prescription for what ails some of America's physicians. But, for patients, it will be just another highly touted panacea that winds up making matters worse.

"Among companies still providing medical coverage for retirees, prescription drugs have had a 'disproportionate impact,' often accounting for half or more of the plans' cost."

Medicare Benefits Should Be Expanded to Cover Prescription Drugs

Patricia Barry

In the following viewpoint, Patricia Barry argues that in addition to the medical benefits provided to Americans over the age of sixty-five by federally funded Medicare, seniors need a drug subsidy to help offset skyrocketing prescription costs. Many companies are cutting back on drug benefits or increasing prescription copayments for retirees, and some no longer offer health coverage to their employees when they retire, according to Barry. Moreover, she maintains, employers would appreciate the relief a Medicare drug benefit would give them to help defray increasing health care costs. Patricia Barry writes about health care issues for the American Association of Retired Persons (AARP).

As you read, consider the following questions:

1. In the author's opinion, what single item contributes most to the increasing cost of health care?
2. According to Barry, what is the "three-tiered" payment system?

The prescription drug crisis in America shows every sign of deepening this year as costs rise and coverage shrinks—not only for most Medicare beneficiaries enrolled in Medicare HMOs but also for many employees and retirees covered by work-based health plans.

In this gloomy climate, The American Association of Retired Persons (AARP) is intensifying its campaign for a Medicare drug benefit, calling on President George W. Bush to revisit the issue in his State of the Union address on January 29, 2002, and to include adequate funding for a benefit in his new budget.

Just a year after Bush came to office promising to make prescription drugs more affordable for older Americans, the issue has taken on a new urgency.

Tax cuts, the vanished surplus and the war on terrorism have all slashed the money available for a drug benefit. At the same time, the problems are getting worse in many segments of society.

As of Jan. 1, 2002, when health plans changed their rates, millions of enrollees are paying a lot more out of pocket for health care.

Sticker shock has hit not only Medicare beneficiaries but also government workers, private-sector employees and companies whose bottom line is being radically affected by the cost of providing health benefits.

"Employers can't continue to absorb record health care premium increases and remain competitive amid the current economic slowdown," said Kate Sullivan, health policy director of the U.S. Chamber of Commerce, in September 2001.

Increasingly, it isn't only consumer groups like AARP that would welcome a Medicare Rx benefit. So too would some of the nation's employers who see it as one way of relieving the pressure of escalating health care inflation.

As vice president of AON Consulting in Wellesley, Massachusetts, Randy Vogenberg advises companies on their prescription drug plans. "What I'm hearing from employers," he says, "is that Medicare drug coverage would certainly help them avoid the difficult decisions they're having to make right now on whether to reduce or eliminate benefits for their own retirees."

Some companies' drug costs remain huge even after cost-saving measures. In January 1993, for example, General Motors (GM) ceased providing direct retiree health benefits for anyone who joined the company after that time. Yet GM still pays out $4 billion a year in health coverage for 500,000 current employees and 700,000 retirees who were working for it before 1993. In 2001—largely because more retirees than active workers are on its health plan—GM spent more than $1 billion of that total on prescription drugs.

"Health care is one of the highest costs in car making," says Robert Minton, GM's health care spokesman.

To sharpen the point, he adds that if any company had $4 billion a year in revenue (instead of health care expenses) it would automatically gain a place on the Fortune 500 list of top-earning companies. "That gives a sense of the magnitude of it," he says.

"This whole health issue—primarily prescription drugs because they contribute to cost increases more than any single thing—is becoming a competitive issue for manufacturers here in the United States," he adds. "It's really affecting our ability to compete on a global basis."

About one-third of Medicare beneficiaries rely on employer-sponsored health plans for drugs.

At present, many of them say that no Medicare proposal yet advanced offers as good a deal as the plan they already have. And they often fear that they may lose retiree Rx benefits if Medicare starts offering one.

But employers' coverage is steadily declining. Only 34 percent of U.S. companies with 200 or more workers offered retiree health benefits in 2001, down from 66 percent in 1988, according to the latest bellwether survey of more than 2,700 companies conducted by the Kaiser Family Foundation research group.

Among companies still providing medical coverage for retirees, prescription drugs have had a "disproportionate impact," often accounting for half or more of the plans' cost, says the Segal Company in its recent survey of 150 such plans nationwide.

The result, it predicted, "is likely to be a significant erosion in privately sponsored retiree health coverage, either through retiree health plan terminations or major changes to plan offerings."

This shrinkage will affect future retirees more than present ones. But the aftershocks of the September 11, 2001, terrorist attacks on America, and the slipping of the economy into recession add to everyone's uncertainty. The news of Polaroid's filing for bankruptcy in October 2001—and immediately cutting off health insurance to its 6,000 retirees—sent more than a few nervous tremors through the retired population.

As health care inflation continues its upward spiral—with prescription drug costs alone expected to rise between 11 and 18 percent in 2002, according to different estimates—something has had to give.

The most common response of health plans is to raise premiums and/or reduce benefits—in other words, transfer more of the burden to the consumer, a practice known as cost shifting.

Premiums are up across the board, in both the private and public sectors. The Federal Employees Health Benefits Program, which covers some 9 million federal workers, retirees and dependents and is often seen as a barometer of health cost trends, has increased premiums by an average 13.3 percent in 2002. The new rates are almost 50 percent higher than five years ago.

Among Medicare HMOs, the average monthly premium rose even more steeply—by 50 percent—from $22 in 2001 to $33 in 2002, according to Medicare statistics.

The number of HMOs offering zero premiums—which first attracted many Medicare beneficiaries to them only a few years ago—is shrinking rapidly, whereas some premiums have shot up to as high as $90 and $150 a month.

In trying to cut their prescription drug costs, both private- and public-sector plans have resorted to a number of strategies.

Over the past few years, the most common has been a switch to the "three-tier" payment system, where enrollees are charged different copayments for different categories of drugs. A typical example: $5 to $10 for generics, $15 for a "preferred" brand name (the brand for which the plan can negotiate the best discount) and $25 for other brand names.

Some plans penalize brand choice more heavily, charging from $40 to $75 in copays for a 30-day supply.

Average Retail Prescription Prices Doubled from 1990 to 2000

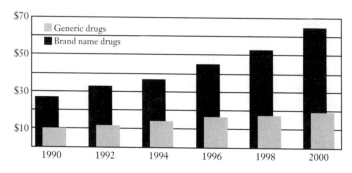

AARP, *AARP Bulletin Online*, March 2002.

Another cost shift requires enrollees to pay a percentage of the cost of the drug instead of a flat copay. Coinsurance of 50 percent or higher is not uncommon. Most plans now offer price incentives to persuade people to choose generics rather than more expensive brand name drugs.

General Motors retirees, for example, can obtain generics for a flat $5 copay. Moreover, the company has embarked on an intensive education campaign to promote the use of generics, at least in part to counteract the impact of the drug manufacturers' heavy advertising of brand names. "For our retirees on a fixed income," says GM's director of pharmacy services, Cynthia Kirman, this policy "can provide more value and maintain quality."

It also saves the company money. In the case of five drugs that have recently been granted patent extensions, GM could have saved "close to $200 million over three years if they had already become available as generics," Kirman says.

With only about half of current drugs available in generic form, the trend toward more expensive copays for brand names pushes up the out-of-pocket costs of many beneficiaries.

Even more restrictive, for some, is the emergence in 2002 of many more plans covering only generic drugs.

More than 1.2 million Medicare beneficiaries—three times as many as last year—now have this limited coverage, though some plans say they will consider covering brand names in cases of "medical necessity."

Such strategies can only work for so long, analysts say. But the prospect of Congress passing any Medicare drug benefit in the coming session—let alone one that would be more attractive to Medicare beneficiaries than past proposals—still appears remote.[1]

"Until Congress makes some decisions it's hard for the private sector to make decisions," says AON's Vogenberg. "You're left with doing stopgap things. Post–September 11, there's been little leadership on this issue. But its such an important issue, it needs to be addressed and resolved."

One event that will dominate political deliberations in 2002 and perhaps persuade lawmakers to focus again on urgent items on the domestic agenda, is the November midterm election.

The Bush administration is already doing its utmost to bring out its promised Medicare drug discount card, which has been delayed by legal issues since September 2001. Medicare chief Thomas Scully has said he hopes the card will be available by spring.

Both he and Health and Human Services Secretary Tommy Thompson insist that the card is no substitute for a prescription drug benefit.

Democrats, who dismiss the card as providing little real help to beneficiaries, nevertheless fear that Republican candidates will use it as evidence of "something done" on prescription drugs in the coming electoral battle for control of Congress.

"The political environment on Capitol Hill is going to be difficult this year," says John Rother, AARP's director of policy. "But Congress needs to address these needs without further delay. And that will require a very strong message from AARP members all over the country."

---

1. As this volume went to press, Congress had not passed a medicare drug benefit.

"The elderly are the most potent voting bloc in America. . . . Therefore, members of Congress give the elderly whatever they want, no matter what the need or the cost."

Medicare Benefits Should Not Be Expanded to Cover Prescription Drugs

Bruce Bartlett

In the following viewpoint, Bruce Bartlett argues that as the wealthiest group in the nation, seniors do not need a prescription drug subsidy in addition to medical benefits from federally funded Medicare. Americans over the age of sixty-five now get more in Social Security benefits than they ever paid in, he maintains. He contends that seniors' power as a voting bloc allows them to manipulate politicians to get whatever they want. According to Bartlett, younger working adults, the majority of whom do not bother to vote, will pay the bill for senior entitlements. Bruce Bartlett is a senior fellow at the National Center for Policy Analysis.

As you read, consider the following questions:
1. What does Bartlett predict will happen when the government starts paying for seniors' prescriptions?
2. In the author's opinion, why are seniors the richest segment of the population?
3. What should taxpayers do to stop senior entitlements, according to the author?

It is now a foregone conclusion that some sort of prescription drug benefit for the elderly will be enacted by Congress and signed into law this year [2001]. The Congressional Budget Office (CBO.) cleared the way for this action on June 11, [2001,] when it estimated the cost of a Senate Democrat plan at just $318 billion over 10 years—close to the $300 billion provided for in the budget. Democrats reportedly were overjoyed at this modest cost estimate, having expected something closer to $400 billion. [As of October 2002, no drug benefit bill had been passed.]

Of course, even $400 billion is probably a very low estimate of the true, ultimate cost of this legislation. It is safe to assume, based on the experience with past entitlement programs, that once implemented the cost of a prescription drug plan inevitably will skyrocket far beyond even the highest projection.

The reason is that estimates never accurately predict how such programs will change behavior. When the government starts paying the bills for prescription drugs, however, we can safely assume that people are going to use a lot more of them. Moreover, the increased demand for drugs will raise their prices above what otherwise would be the case.

Seniors Do Not Need a Drug Benefit

But there is a larger question about this legislation and that is, Why enact it at all? There is really no demonstrable need for it. The answer is that the elderly are the most potent voting bloc in America. For example, in the 1998 congressional elections, just 42 percent of all registered voters voted, but almost 60 percent of those over age 65 did. Therefore, members of Congress give the elderly whatever they want, no matter what the need or the cost.

Contributing to Congress's incentive to pander shamelessly to every whim of the elderly is the fact that those who pay the bills for such pandering barely vote at all. Among those between the ages of 18 and 24, who will end up paying through the nose for the prescription drug plan, only 16.6 percent voted in 1998, according to the Census Bureau. In short, you cannot really blame politicians when they can freely take money from those who don't vote and use it to buy votes from those who do.

This is grossly unfair. Just because some people allow themselves to be taken advantage of doesn't make it right to do so, nor is it right to pander to the politically powerful just because it works. This is especially the case when those who are being taken advantage of are relatively poor and those who are being pandered to are far better off financially.

There Is Little Interest in Prescription Insurance

Most Medicare beneficiaries are more interested in getting someone else to guarantee them lower drug prices (or pay most of their bills) than in purchasing "insurance" protection at market-based prices. A recent survey of seniors conducted by Harvard's Kennedy School of Government found that 7 out of 10 seniors would personally be willing to pay no more than $30 a month ($360 a year) for prescription drug coverage that paid for at least half of their prescription drug bills (roughly a $640 net subsidy, given that the survey assumed the average senior's annual prescription drug costs are $2000). Thirty percent said they would not be willing to pay anything at all for such subsidized drug coverage.

Tom Miller, *FOX News Online*, July 18, 2002.

The fact is that the elderly are the wealthiest group in American society and the least deserving of more government hand-outs. They already receive vastly more in Social Security benefits than any of them ever paid in to the system, with the difference being taxed from today's workers. Nor do the elderly pay more than a tiny fraction of the cost of Medicare. It is essentially a welfare program for anyone over age 65, no matter how well off they may be.

Seniors Are Healthy and Wealthy

Increasingly the elderly are rich, in large part because they don't have to pay for things that the working population has to pay for, such as health care.

• According to a recent Census Bureau report, those age 65 to 69 have the highest median net worth of any age group: $106,408 in 1995.

• By contrast, those under age 35 had a net worth of just

$7,428, and those between the ages of 35 and 44 had a net worth of only $31,691.

A prime source of the elderly's growing wealth is that many own their homes free and clear. According to the Bureau of Labor Statistics, 65.4 percent of elderly homeowners in 1997 had no mortgage. Therefore, they had no mortgage payment and paid no rent. Yet many still have substantial incomes from pensions and investments, as well as Social Security.

• According to a new study from the CBO, the average after-tax income of elderly households is just 10 percent less than that of the nonelderly: $44,000 for the former and $48,500 for the latter.

• When one takes into account Medicare and the value of assets, it turns out that the elderly as a group are 24 percent better off than the nonelderly, according to a study by economists Stephen Crystal and Dennis Shea, both of Rutgers University.

• They further estimate that the elderly are 83 percent better off than families with small children.

These conclusions are not disputed by advocates for the elderly. A new American Association of Retired People (AARP) report, *Beyond 50*, shows that the elderly as a whole have never been wealthier or healthier.

Nevertheless, the view persists in many circles that the elderly are overwhelmingly poor and in ill health. That is what justifies the enactment of ever more give-away programs for them by Congress. Unfortunately, it will continue until those who are taxed to pay the bills finally demand fairness and start voting in larger numbers to get it.

Periodical Bibliography

The following articles have been selected to supplement the diverse views presented in this chapter.

Jonathan Alter	"Fighting the HMO Meanies: Managed Care Is the Only Industry in America That Can't Be Sued. That Makes No Sense," *Newsweek*, August 6, 2001.
American Association of Retired Persons	"Medicare Prescription Drugs: Just the Facts," September 28, 2002. www.aarp.org.
American Medical News	"The Privacy Balancing Act," March 20, 2000, www.ama-assn.org.
Joseph Antos, Grace-Marie Turner, and Robert E. Moffit	"Time for a Sensible Medicare Drug Benefit," American Institute for Public Policy, *Articles*, August 30, 2002.
LaCrisha Butler	"How to Cover Medicare Drugs," *American Medical News*, March 13, 2000.
Fred H. Cate	"Principles for Protecting Privacy," *Cato Journal*, Spring/Summer 2002.
Tom A. Coburn	"Patients' Rights, Done Wrong," *New York Times*, July 30, 1999.
Jamie Court	"Reforming HMOs While Deforming Our Beleaguered Tort System," *San Diego Union-Tribune*, August 25, 1999.
Michael Jonathan Grinfeld	"Will Physicians' Unions Destroy the Medical Profession?" *Medicine & Behavior*, December 1998. www.medicineandbehavior.com.
Dick Meister	"An Essential Rx for Tomorrow's Doctors," *LaborNet*, May 2000. www.labornet.org.
Susan Harrington Preston	"Doctor Unions, Time to Join the Parade?" *Medical Economics*, January 24, 2000. www.memag.com.
Robert J. Samuelson	"It's More Than a Drug Problem: Expanding Medicare Would Force Tomorrow's Workers to Subsidize Baby Boomers' Retirement," *Newsweek*, September 25, 2000.
Texas Conservative Coalition	"Six Cautions on Expanding Medical Liability," *Lift Perspective*, February 18, 2000. www.txccri.org.
L. Samuel Wann	"A Union of Doctors?" *American College of Cardiology Web Editorial*, August 1999. www.acc.org.

Glossary

adverse selection The tendency of persons who present a poorer-than-average health risk to apply for, or continue, insurance to a greater extent than do persons with average or better-than-average expectations of health.

benefit package The covered services each patient is entitled to under a **managed care** contract.

capitation An arrangement in which **managed care** plans pay a fixed monthly or annual fee to physicians for each patient in their care. Doctors receive the same fixed amount each month regardless of how much care the plan member receives.

claim A request by either an individual or his or her physician asking an insurance company to pay for services the insured obtained from a health care professional.

copayment The percentage or proportion of a health insurance **claim** that is paid directly "out of pocket" by the patient.

deductible The fixed amount of money that an individual must pay before the insurance company will begin to reimburse for services.

fee-for-service The traditional way of paying for medical services. Doctors in private practice charge a fee for each service provided, and the patient's insurer pays all or part of that fee.

gatekeeper A health care professional (usually a physician) responsible for coordinating a patient's utilization of services and controlling access to specialists and procedures. The primary purpose of having a gatekeeper is to control costs and prevent unnecessary utilization of services.

health maintenance organization (HMO) A **managed care** plan that provides health care in return for preset monthly payments. Physicians in these plans share in the financial risk for the delivery of health services, and enrollees typically are not covered to see physicians who do not have a contract with the HMO.

managed care A variety of health care financing and delivery systems that are designed to limit costs and control use of health care services. Some managed care plans attempt to improve health quality by emphasizing prevention of disease.

Medicaid A combined federally- and state-funded program that provides health care for the indigent population (individuals living below the poverty line). Medicaid was established in 1965 under the Social Security Act to help reduce the number of uninsured Americans.

Medicare A federal entitlement program that provides health care benefits to individuals who are over sixty-five years of age, blind, disabled, or have renal disease. Medicare Part A provides coverage for hospital visits and Medicare Part B provides physician visits, pharmacy, and other health services. Medicare is an entitlement program—everybody who falls into one of the previously mentioned categories automatically receives benefits. However, individuals who receive Medicare must pay **deductibles**,

premiums, and **copayments** to receive services. Medicare was established in 1965 as part of the Social Security Act.

outpatient   A patient who receives health care services (such as surgery) on an outpatient basis, meaning they do not stay overnight in a hospital or inpatient facility. Many insurance companies have identified a list of tests and procedures (including surgery) that will not be covered (paid for) unless they are performed on an outpatient basis.

point-of-service option   A provision in some **HMO** contracts that allows patients to choose to pay extra in order to have the **HMO** provide coverage for services rendered by physicians who are not included in the health plan's network.

preexisting condition   A medical condition that is excluded from coverage by an insurance company because the condition was believed to exist prior to the individual's obtaining a policy from the particular insurance company.

premium   The (usually monthly) sum paid by a policyholder to keep his or her insurance policy in force.

primary care physician   *See* **gatekeeper**

provider   Any health professional who provides medical-related services. This broader term is often used in place of *doctor* or *physician* to encompass registered nurses, therapists, hospitals, dentists, etc.

third-party payment   Payment of medical services by an entity other than the individual receiving the services or the **provider** of the services. An example of third-party payment is reimbursement by an insurance company or the federal government through the **Medicare** program to a doctor or hospital. The third party is not directly involved with the delivery of service.

For Further Discussion

Chapter 1

1. Authors at the Bureau of Labor Education at the University of Maine point to low scores on a recent World Health Organization (WHO) survey as proof that Americans are paying too much and getting too little in the way of health care. Which of WHO's three goals (the provision of good health, responsiveness to the expectations of the population, and the fairness of the individuals' financial contribution toward their health care) do you think is most important to Americans. Why?

2. More than 40 million Americans lack health insurance. Tom Miller maintains that they do not need it and will not suffer medically or financially if they do not have it. Lisa Climan and Adria Scharf provide the stories of people who are suffering because they do not have insurance. Who makes the better case? How do Miller's studies and statistics stand up against Climan and Scharf's real people?

3. Mick L. Diede and Richard Liliedahl maintain that health care spending is out of control and must be brought into line by sacrifices of all health care system players. Charles R. Morris says that increasing health care spending is a good thing because it puts money back into the economy. In your opinion, which author makes the most convincing argument? Why?

Chapter 2

1. Edmund D. Pellegrino maintains that where health care is concerned, ethics must always take precedence over economics. Is it acceptable, then, for a doctor to lie to her patient's HMO in order to ensure that necessary procedures for the patient are covered? Explain.

2. Larry Van Heerden argues that health care is just like any other product or service and that supply and demand should be determined by the marketplace. Do you agree? Why or why not?

3. Karlyn Bowman says that the poor opinion most people have of managed care results from media exaggerations and friends' horror stories rather than their own positive experiences. Why do you think people would place more weight on what they see in movies and on television than in their own personal experiences?

Chapter 3

1. Robert L. Ferrer provides an emotional argument for universal health care when he writes in detail about the terrible medical

and social conditions of uninsured Americans. L. Dean Forman practically argues that, from a financial and political point of view, universal health care would be a disaster. Which author do you think offers the most persuasive argument? Why?

2. Jeff Lemieux insists that tax credits are necessary because they help provide health insurance, and therefore access to health care, for the uninsured. Tom Miller argues that tax credits reinforce the concept of entitlements and should not be allowed because health insurance is not required to access health care. Which author is more convincing? Why?

3. Harry M.J. Kraemer Jr., Sara J. Singer, and Jerry Geisel each offer a different solution to the problem of uninsured Americans. While the solutions share common elements, each is unique and would require substantial changes to the current U.S. health care system. Which author makes the strongest argument for his or her concept as a viable solution? Explain.

Chapter 4

1. David Orentlicher argues that medical IDs would improve health care and maintains that strict safeguards would ensure privacy. Maggie Scarf contends that potential loss of personal privacy outweighs any positives that might result from medical IDs. After examining the evidence that each author provides, which do you think makes the most convincing argument? Explain.

2. Patients, doctors, lawyers, and health care organizations all have a stake in the HMO liability debate. William B. Schwartz argues that patients and their HMOs will benefit. Richard A. Epstein contends that HMOs will suffer and so will patients. Who do you think has the most to gain if patients are allowed to sue their HMOs? Who has the most to lose?

3. Glenn Flores argues that doctors want to unionize because it will give them more power as patient advocates, and he claims that physicians would never go on strike. Joshua M. Sharfstein contends that doctors are really trying to unionize to better their own financial and social status. Who do you think offers the stronger argument? Explain.

4. Bruce Bartlett maintains that the majority of seniors are wealthy and do not need help with the cost of prescription drugs. On the other hand, Patricia Barry insists that a Medicare drug benefit is the only option for the less well off elderly who may have no other retirement benefits or are losing the ones they do have. Who makes a stronger argument?

Organizations to Contact

The editors have compiled the following list of organizations concerned with the issues debated in this book. The descriptions are derived from materials provided by the organizations. All have publications or information available for interested readers. The list was compiled on the date of publication of the present volume; the information provided here may change. Be aware that many organizations take several weeks or longer to respond to inquiries, so allow as much time as possible.

American Association of Retired Persons (AARP)
601 E St. NW, Washington, DC 20049
(800) 424-3410
website: www.aarp.org

AARP is a nonprofit, nonpartisan membership organization for people 50 and over. It provides information and resources; advocates on legislative, consumer, and legal issues; assists members to serve their communities; and offers a wide range of unique benefits, special products, and services for members. These benefits include AARP Webplace at www.aarp.org, *AARP Modern Maturity* and *My Generation* magazines, the monthly *AARP Bulletin*, and a Spanishlanguage newspaper, *Segunda Juventud*. Active in every state, the District of Columbia, Puerto Rico, and the U.S. Virgin Islands, AARP celebrates the attitude that age is just a number and life is what you make it.

American Enterprise Institute (AEI)
1150 17th St. NW, Washington, DC 20036
(202) 862-5800 • fax: (202) 862-7178
website: www.aei.org

The American Enterprise Institute for Public Policy Research is dedicated to preserving and strengthening the foundations of freedom—limited government, private enterprise, vital cultural and political institutions, and a strong foreign policy and national defense—through scholarly research, open debate, and publications. Founded in 1943, AEI researches economics and trade; social welfare and health; government tax, spending, regulatory, and legal policies; U.S. politics; international affairs; and U.S. defense and foreign policies. The institute publishes dozens of books and hundreds of articles and reports each year and a policy magazine, the *American Enterprise*.

American Society of Law, Medicine & Ethics (ASLME)
765 Commonwealth Ave., Suite 1634, Boston, MA 02215
(617) 262-4990 • fax: (617) 437-7596
e-mail: info@aslme.org • website: www.aslme.org

The mission of ASLME is to provide high-quality scholarship, debate, and critical thought to professionals in the fields of law, health care, policy, and ethics. The society acts as a source of guidance and information through the publication of two quarterlies, the *Journal of Law, Medicine & Ethics* and the *American Journal of Law & Medicine*.

Brookings Institution
1775 Massachusetts Ave. NW, Washington, DC 20036-2188
(202) 797-6105 • fax: (202) 797-2495
website: www.brook.edu

Founded in 1927, the institution is a liberal research and education organization that publishes material on economics, government, and foreign policy. It strives to serve as a bridge between scholarship and public policy, bringing new knowledge to the attention of decision makers and providing scholars with improved insight into public policy issues. The Brookings Institution produces hundreds of abstracts and reports on health care with topics ranging from Medicaid to persons with disabilities.

Cato Institute
1000 Massachusetts Ave. NW, Washington, DC 20001-5403
(202) 842-0200 • fax: (202) 842-3490
e-mail: cato@cato.org • website: www.cato.org

The institute is a libertarian public policy research foundation dedicated to limiting the role of government and protecting individual liberties. Its Health and Welfare Studies department works to formulate and popularize a free-market agenda for health care reform. The institute publishes the quarterly magazine *Regulation*, the bimonthly *Cato Policy Report*, and numerous books and commentaries, hundreds of which relate to health care.

Center for Studying Health System Change (HSC)
600 Maryland Ave. SW, #550, Washington, DC 20024
(202) 484-5261 • fax: (202) 484-9258
website: www.hschange.com

The Center for Studying Health System Change is a nonpartisan policy research organization. HSC designs and conducts studies focused on the U.S. health care system to inform the thinking and decisions of policy makers in government and private industry. In addition to this applied use, HSC studies contribute more broadly to the body of health care policy research that enables decision makers to understand changes to the health care system and the national and local market forces driving those changes. They publish issue briefs, community reports, tracking reports, data bulletins, and journal articles based on their research.

Healthcare Leadership Council (HLC)

900 17th St. NW, Suite 600, Washington, DC 20006
(202) 452-8700
website: www.hlc.org

The council is a forum in which health care industry leaders can jointly develop policies, plans, and programs that support a market-based health care system. HLC believes America's health care system should value innovation and provide affordable high-quality health care free from excessive government regulations. It offers the latest press releases on health issues and several public policy papers with titles such as "Empowering Consumers and Patients" and "Ensuring Responsible Government."

Heritage Foundation

214 Massachusetts Ave. NE, Washington, DC 20002-4999
(800) 544-4843 • (202) 546-4400 • fax: (202) 544-6979
e-mail: pubs@heritage.org • website: www.heritage.org

The foundation is a public policy research institute that advocates limited government and the free market system. It believes the private sector, not government, should be relied upon to ease social problems. The Heritage Foundation publishes the quarterly *Policy Review*, as well as hundreds of monographs, books, and background papers with titles such as *Medicare Minus Choice* and *What to Do About Uninsured Children*.

Institute for Health Freedom (IHF)

1825 Eye St. NW, Washington, DC 20036
(202) 429-6610 • fax: (202) 861-1973
website: www.forhealthfreedom.org

The institute is a nonpartisan, nonprofit research center established to bring the issues of personal freedom in choosing health care to the forefront of America's health policy debate. Its mission is to present the ethical and economic case for strengthening personal health freedom. IHF's research and analyses are published as policy briefings, including "Children's Health Care," "Monopoly in Medicine," and "Legal Issues." All are available through its website.

National Center for Policy Analysis (NCPA)
655 15th St. NW, Suite 375, Washington, DC 20005
(202) 628-6671 • fax: (202) 628-6474
e-mail: ncpa@public-policy.org • website: www.ncpa.org

NCPA is a nonprofit public policy research institute. It publishes the bimonthly newsletter *Executive Alert* as well as numerous health care policy studies, including "Saving Medicare" and "Medical Savings Accounts: Obstacles to Their Growth and Ways to Improve Them," and its website includes an extensive section on health care issues.

National Coalition on Health Care
1200 G St. NW, Suite 750, Washington, DC 20005
(202) 638-7151 • fax: (202) 638-7166
website: www.nchc.org

The National Coalition on Health Care is a nonprofit, nonpartisan group that represents the nation's largest alliance working to improve America's health care and make it more affordable. The coalition offers several policy studies including "Why the Quality of U.S. Health Care Must Be Improved" and "The Rising Number of Uninsured Workers: An Approaching Crisis in Health Care Financing."

Urban Institute
2100 M St. NW, Washington, DC 20037
(202) 261-5244
website: www.urban.org

The Urban Institute investigates social and economic problems confronting the nation and analyzes efforts to solve these problems. In addition, the institute works to improve government decisions and to increase citizen awareness about important public choices. It offers a wide variety of resources, including books such as *Restructuring Medicare: Impacts on Beneficiaries* and *The Decline in Medical Spending Growth in 1996: Why Did It Happen?*

Bibliography of Books

George Anders — *Health Against Wealth: HMOs and the Breakdown of Medical Trust.* Thorndike, ME: G.K. Hall, 1997.

Sue Blevins — *Medicare's Midlife Crisis.* Washington, DC: CATO, 2001.

Grace Burdrys and Gladys Burdrys — *Our Unsystematic Health Care System.* Lanham, MD: Rowan and Littlefield, 2001.

Grace Burdrys and Gladys Burdrys — *When Doctors Join Unions.* Ithaca, NY: ILP Press/Cornell University Press, 1997.

Lawton R. Burns — *The Health Care Value Chain: Producers, Purchasers, and Providers.* San Francisco: Jossey-Bass, 2002.

Jamie Court, ed. — *Making a Killing: HMOs and the Threat to Your Health.* Monroe, ME: Common Courage Press, 1999.

David Dranove — *The Economic Evolution of American Health Care.* Princeton, NJ: Princeton University Press, 2000.

Sherry Glied — *Chronic Condition: Why Health Reform Fails.* Cambridge, MA: Harvard University Press, 1997.

Martin L. Gross — *The Medical Racket: How Doctors, HMOs, and Hospitals Are Failing the American Patient.* New York: Avon Books, 1998.

Robert B. Hackey — *Rethinking Health Care Policy: The New Politics of State Regulation.* Washington, DC: Georgetown University Press, 1998.

Charlene Harrington and Carroll L. Estes, eds. — *Health Policy: Crisis and Reform in the U.S. Health Care Delivery System.* Sudbury, MA: Jones and Bartlett, 2001.

Regina E. Herzlinger — *Market-Driven Healthcare: Who Wins, Who Loses in the Transformation of America's Largest Service Industry.* Reading, MA: Perseus, 1999.

Institute for the Future — *Health and Health Care 2010.* San Francisco: Jossey-Bass, 2000.

Paul Jesilow, Henry N. Pontell, and Gilbert Geis — *Prescription for Profit: How Doctors Defraud Medicare.* Berkeley: University of California Press, 1993.

J.D. Kleinke — *Oxymorons: The Myth of a U.S. Health Care System.* San Francisco: Jossey-Bass, 2001.

Melvin J. Konner — *Medicine at the Crossroads: The Crisis in Health Care.* New York: Vintage Books, 1994.

George D. Lundberg and James H. Stacey — *Severed Trust: Why American Medicine Hasn't Been Fixed.* Denver, CO: Basic Books, 2001.

Michael Marmot and Richard Wilkinson, eds. — *Social Determinants of Health.* New York: Oxford University Press, 1999.

David Mechanic — *Mental Health and Social Policy: The Emergence of Managed Care.* Boston: Allyn and Bacon, 1998.

Michael L. Millenson — *Demanding Medical Excellence: Doctors and Accountability in the Information Age.* Chicago: University of Chicago Press, 1997.

Robert I. Misbin — *Health Care Crisis: The Search for Answers.* Frederick, MD: University Publishing Group, 1995.

Rudolph J. Mueller — *As Sick As It Gets: The Shocking Reality of America's Healthcare: A Diagnosis and Treatment Plan.* Dunkirk, NY: Olin Frederick, 2001.

Lawrence J. O'Brien — *Bad Medicine: How the American Medical Establishment Is Ruining Our Healthcare System.* Amherst, NY: Prometheus Books, 1999.

Kant Patel and Mark Rushefsky — *Health Care Politics and Policy in America.* Armonk, NY: M.E. Sharpe, 1999.

Mark V. Pauly — *An Analysis of Medical Savings Accounts: Do Two Wrongs Make a Right?* Washington, DC: AEI Press, 1994.

Molly Shapiro — *What You Need to Know About HMOs and the Patient's Bill of Rights.* Freedom, CA: Crossing Press, 1999.

David G. Smith — *Entitlement Politics: Medicare and Medicaid, 1995–2001.* New York: Aldine de Gruyter, 2002.

Mickey C. Smith — *Prescription Drugs Under Medicare: The Legacy of the Task Force on Prescription Drugs.* New York: Pharmaceutical Products Press, 2001.

Thomas Szasz — *Pharmacracy: Medicine and Politics in America.* Westport, CT: Praeger, 2001.

E. Fuller Torrey — *Out of the Shadows: Confronting America's Mental Illness Crisis.* New York: John Wiley, 1997.

Carol S. Weissert and William G. Weissert — *Governing Health: The Politics of Health Policy.* Baltimore: Johns Hopkins University Press, 1996.

Howard Wolinsky and Tom Brune — *The Serpent on the Staff: The Unhealthy Politics of the American Medical Association.* New York: G.P. Putnam's Sons, 1994.

Lisa Yount — *Patients' Rights in the Age of Managed Care.* New York: Facts On File, 2001.

Index

ABC News poll, 101
Ad Hoc Committee to Defend Health Care, 90–91
Adler, Nancy, 40
advertising
  of prescription drugs, 15
  costs of, 14
Aetna
  vs. Louisville doctors, 195–97
Altman, Stuart, 92
American Association of Retired Persons (AARP), 199, 207
American Medical Association, 191
Anderson, William L., 15
Appelbaum, Paul, 179
Armey, Dick, 130

Barry, Patricia, 198
Bartlett, Bruce, 204
Beyond 50 (American Association of Retired Persons), 207
Bowman, Karlyn, 100
Brandeis, Louis D., 10
Brook, Robert, 85
Bureau of Labor Education at the University of Maine, 23
Bureau of Labor Statistics, 207
Burgess, Michael, 156
Bush, George W., 80, 130, 165, 194
  promise for Medicare prescription benefit by, 199
  tax credit proposals of, 134
    flaws in, 129, 152
Business Insurance (magazine), 154
Butler, Stuart, 137

Califano, Joseph A., Jr., 16
California Public Employees Retirement System (CalPERS), 148
Canada
  rationing of health care in, 124
Care Without Coverage: Too Little, Too Late (Institute of Medicine), 39
charity care, 112–13
Cigna Corporation, 69
Climan, Lisa, 33
Clinton, Bill, 57, 81, 82, 104
  opposition to health care reform by, 106
Clinton, Hillary, 81
Congressional Budgeting Office (CBO)
  on after-tax income of elderly households, 207
  on increases in premiums, 55

on single-payer plan, 32
Consolidated Omnibus Budget Reconciliation Act (COBRA), 49, 118, 133, 134
Consumers Union, 135
Costello, Kit, 118
cost-sharing
  reduces use of medical services, 97–99
Crystal, Stephen, 207
Cunningham, Peter J., 112

Davis, Gray, 122
Decade of the Brain, 164, 165
default plans, 150
Denenberg, Herb, 182
Department of Health and Human Services, U.S., 168
Diede, Mick L., 47
Dingell, John, 185
direct-to-consumer (DTC) marketing, 14–15
  impact of, on health care system, 15
disability-adjusted life expectancy (DALE)
  in U.S., vs. high-income OECD countries, 28, 29
Domenici, Peter, 164

Easterbrook, Gregg, 79
education, 44–45
elderly
  are healthy and wealthy, 206–207
  do not need prescription drug benefits, 205–206
  growth in population of, 11
Ellwood, Paul, 68, 69, 160
Employee Retirement Income Security Act (ERISA), 182
employer-based insurance
  is best answer for the uninsured, 138–46
  prevalence of, 143
Enthoven, Alain C., 68, 69, 148
Epstein, Richard A., 184
evidence-based medicine, 63–64
Exploring the Health-Wealth Nexus (Meer and Rosen), 43

Federal Employees Health Benefits (FEHB) Program, 148, 149
  increase in costs to, 201
fee-for-service programs
  vs. managed care, health outcomes in, 85–86

Ferrer, Robert L., 114
Financial Impact of Health Insurance, The (Levy), 46
First American Conference on Social Insurance (1913), 10
Fisher, Elliott, 43
Flexner, Abraham, 18
Flores, Glenn, 189
Food and Drug Administration (FDA), 18
Forman, L. Dean, 121
Fox, Nelene, 87
Frist, William H., 19

Garber, Alan, 148
Geisel, Jerry, 154
General Accounting Office (GAO)
  on single-payer plan, 32
General Motors
  health coverage expenditures by, 200
  prescription drug coverage by, 202
Glied, Sherry, 58, 59, 60
Goldman, Dana, 44
Goodman, Ellen, 14
Gore, Al, 130, 174
Gostin, Larry, 175
government
  role of, in health plan oversight, 102–103
Grealy, Mary R., 142

Haas, Jennifer, 40
Hadley, Jack, 40–41
Hand, Learned, 181
Harding, Richard K., 175
Hart, Julian Tudor, 117
Hazlett, Thomas W., 89
health, status of
  vs. health care utilization, as measures of outcome, 40
  indicators of, 27–28
    in high-income OECD countries, 28
  link with education, 44–45
  link with socioeconomic status, 41–42
Health Across America campaign, 139–40
Health Affairs (journal), 43
health care
  financing
    fairness in, 30
    reform of, as best answer for uninsured, 147–53
  is a minor fraction of total economy, 59
  market-driven solutions to, 96–97
  myth of nonproductivity of, 60–61

spending
  containment crisis is overstated, 62
  increase in, 64–65, 107–108
  is a serious problem, 47–55
    con, 56–65
  managed care is necessary to control, 81–82, 89–92
    con, 93–99
  per capita
    estimates of rise in, 48, 51
    in high-income OECD countries, 26
    in U.S., 25–26
system
  indicators of, in high-income OECD countries, 28
  managed care has harmed, 70–78
    con, 79–88
  medical IDs would improve, 166–72
    con, 173–79
  mergers and acquisitions in, 69
  satisfaction with, in U.S. vs. other countries, 31
  uninsured suffer most in, 115–17
  in U.S., is best in the world, 16–22
    con, 23–32
  utilization of, vs. health status as measure of outcomes, 40
Healthcare Leadership Council (HLC), 139
Health Employer Data Information System (HEDIS), 84
Health Insurance Portability and Accountability Act (1996), 54
Health Maintenance Organization Assistance Act (1973), 68
health maintenance organizations (HMOs), 68
  average increase in rates of, 50
  costs to administer, 125–26
  denial of care by, can cause injury/death, 190–91
  executive compensation in, 192
  increase in monthly premiums of, 201–202
  lawsuits would be disastrous for, 184–88
    con, 180–83
  participation in, 68–69
  patients' rights legislation and, 80
  patients should be allowed to sue, 180–83
    con, 184–88
  survey on patient satisfaction with, 101–102, 103
  see also managed care
Herdrich, Cindy, 80, 85, 86, 87

HMOs. *See* health maintenance
  organizations

infant mortality
  in U.S. vs. high-income OECD
    countries, 28, 29
informed consent
  medical IDs are a threat to, 179
  Institute of Medicine (IOM), 39
insurance, health
  affordability is key to coverage,
    148–50
  health status and, no causal
    relationship has been found
    between, 46
  is not an entitlement, 136–37
  tax credits should be used to expand
    coverage, 127–31
    con, 132–37
  see also uninsured individuals
*Insurance and the Utilization of Medical
  Services Among the Self-Employed*
  (Rosen and Perry), 45
insurance exchanges, 149
*In Their Own Words: The Uninsured
  Talk About Living Without Health
  Insurance* (Kaiser Commission on
  Medicaid and the Uninsured), 34

Jacobs, Andy, 156
Johnson, Lyndon B., 10, 20

Kaiser Commission on Medicaid and
  the Uninsured, 34
Kaiser Family Foundation, 40, 200
Kaiser Family Foundation/Harvard
  survey, 102–103
Kaiser Permanente, 106, 109
Kane, Carol K., 113
Kelber, Harry, 191
Kennedy-Kassebaum Health Insurance
  Policy Act (1996), 167, 174
Kirman, Cynthia, 202–203
Klein, Joel, 195
Kraemer, Harry M.J., Jr., 138

Lakdawalla, Darius, 44
Larsen, Robert R., 187
lawsuits
  cost is not the issue in, 182
    con, 187
  negligence must be proven in,
    181–82
  would be disastrous for HMOs,
    184–88
    con, 180–83
Lazarus, Ian R., 91
Lemieux, Jeff, 127

Lesch, Michael, 60, 63
Levy, Helen, 46
life expectancy. *See* disability-adjusted
  life expectancy
Liliedahl, Richard, 47
Lleras-Muney, Adriana, 44–45
LoBuono, Charlotte, 84
Los Angeles Times (newspaper), 179

managed care
  controls cost by negotiating
    discounts, 82–83
  discourages innovative technology,
    78
  ethical issues in, 71
  forces efficiency in health care,
    86–88
  has harmed health care system,
    70–78
    con, 79–88
  is necessary to control health care
    costs, 89–92
    con, 93–99
  most patients are satisfied with,
    100–104
    con, 50, 105–109
  non-dollar costs affecting quality of,
    77
  rules and red tape contribute to poor
    image of, 83–85
  see also health maintenance
    organizations
McGlynn, Elizabeth, 85
McGuire, William, 192
Meara, Ellen, 41
Medicaid
  establishment of, 10, 20
  as single-payer program, 123
  medical IDs
    strict safeguards would be required,
      171–72
    would improve health care system,
      166–72
      con, 173–79
  medical research
    medical IDs would benefit, 169–70
    U.S. is leader in, 19
  medical savings accounts (MSAs),
    95–96
    are best answer for the uninsured,
      154–61
    flow chart for set up of, 159
    public lacks information about,
      160–61
    satisfaction with, 157–58
Medicare
  benefits should be expanded to cover
    prescription drugs, 198–203

con, 204–207
costs to administer, 125
establishment of, 10, 20
has been a success, 22
issues in debate over, 11
percent spent on last year of life by, 60
pressures for reform of, 12
as single-payer program, 123
ways to improve, 145–46
Meer, Jonathan, 43
Meltzer, David, 46
Mental Health Parity Act (1996), 164, 165
MetraHealth Companies, Inc., 69
Miller, Tom, 38, 132, 206
Minton, Robert, 200
Morris, Charles R., 56
Morris, Scott, 112–13
Murphy, Kevin, 85

National Cancer Institute, 20
National Institutes of Health, 20
National Journal, 101, 104
negligence
must be proven in lawsuits, 181–82
Nelson, Patricia, 35–36
Nelson, William, 35
New England Journal of Medicine, 177
Newhouse, Joseph F., 62
Newman, Russ, 165
New York Post (newspaper), 178
New York Times (newspaper), 194
Nichols, George, III, 196, 197
Nixon, Richard M., 20, 68
Norwood, Charlie, 185
Norwood-Dingell bill, 185

opinion polls. *See* surveys
Orentlicher, David, 166

patient-rights legislation, 55, 80, 107
Pellegrino, Edmund D., 70
Perry, Craig, 45, 137
pharmaceutical companies
advertising by, 14–15
opinion on, 52
Phillips, Andrew, 105
physicians
generalists vs. specialists, 77–78
have moral duty to deny unneeded treatment, 72
HMOs limit earnings of, 91
in Louisville, vs. Aetna, 195–97
in managed care systems
are sometimes forced to lie, 74–75
dilemma of divided loyalty among, 73–74

pressures on, 21
strict rules inhibit, 191–92
numbers providing indigent care, 112
as patient advocates, 75
should be allowed to unionize, 189–92
con, 193–97
surveys of
on prescriptions and DTC marketing, 15
on prevalence of providing indigent care, 112
population, aging of U.S., 11
prescription drugs
direct-to-consumer marketing of, 14–15
Medicare benefits should be expanded to cover, 198–203
con, 204–207
rise in prices for, 202
preventive care, 84
privacy
medical IDs would enhance, 170–71
con, 176–77
role of government in enforcing, 99
Progressive Policy Institute (PPI), 128
Public Health Service, 19
Pyles, Robert, 177

Raible, Robert, 108
Reed, Marie C., 112
Reich, Robert, 61
Relationship Between Education and Adult Mortality in the United States, The (Lleras-Muney), 45
Reschovsky, James D., 103
research. *See* medical research
Roberts, Marc, 91
Roberts, Tom, 36–37
Robinson, James C., 97
Rooney, J. Patrick, 154
Roper Starch Worldwide survey, 101
Rosen, Harvey, 43, 45, 137
Rosenberg, Harry, 85
Rother, John, 203
Ruskin, Jill, 108–109
Ruskin, Paul, 106, 108, 109

Samuelson, Robert J., 42
Scarf, Maggie, 173
Scharf, Adria, 33
Schuster, Mark, 85
Schwartz, William B., 180
Scully, Thomas, 203
seniors. *See* elderly
Shalala, Donna, 174, 175
Sharfstein, Joshua M., 193

Shea, Dennis, 207
Sicker and Poorer: The Consequences of Being Uninsured (Kaiser Family Foundation), 40
Singer, Sara J., 147
single-payer plan
  could be the answer for health care reform, 31–32
  problems with, 95
Skinner, Jonathan, 43
Smith, Ken, 90
Smith, Yolanda, 34–35
Smoak, Randolph D., Jr., 194
Social Security Act (1935), 11
  Title XVIII and Title XIX, 10
socioeconomic status, 41–42
Stark, Pete, 130
State Children's Health Improvement Program (S-CHIP), 139, 140
  ways to improve, 145–46
Stoddard, Jeffery, 112
Sullivan, Kate, 199
Surgeon General's Report on Mental Health in America (1999), 164
surveys
  on decline in employee coverage, 200
  on patient satisfaction with HMOs, 101
  of physicians
    on prescriptions and DTC marketing, 15
    on prevalence of providing indigent care, 112, 113

tax credits
  should be used to expand health insurance coverage, 127–31, 140, 144–45, 149–53
    con, 132–37
Thompson, Tommy, 203
Topel, Robert, 85
Truman, Harry S., 10–11

Understanding Health Disparities Against Education Groups (Goldman and Lakdawalla), 44
uninsured individuals
  employer-based solutions are best answer for, 138–46
  expanding coverage is not the only way to improve health of, 46
  medical savings accounts are best

  answer for, 154–61
  numbers of
    turning down/not offered employer-provided insurance, 141
    in U.S., 27, 34, 81, 109, 151
  profile of, 34
  suffer most in the health care system, 115–17
  universal health care is best solution for, 114–20
    con, 121–26
  in U.S., is a serious problem, 33–37
    con, 38–46
unions
  physicians should be allowed to form, 189–92
    con, 193–97
  professional membership in, is growing, 191
United States
  has best health care system in the world, 16–22
    con, 23–32
  is a leader in medical research, 19
universal health care
  is best solution for uninsured Americans, 114–20
    con, 121–26
  is no panacea, 42
  tax credits are a path to, 129–31

Van Heerden, Larry, 93
Velazquez, Nydia, 178
Vladeck, Bruce, 60
Vogenberg, Randy, 199, 203

Washington Post (newspaper), 130
Weingarten, Scott, 63
Welch, Charles, 179
Wellstone, Paul, 164
Wennberg, John, 43
What Do We Really Know About Whether Health Insurance Affects Health? (Levy and Meltzer), 46
Why Is Health Related to Socioeconomic Status? The Case of Pregnancy and Low Birth Weight (Meara), 41
Woodward, Beverly, 178
World Health Organization (WHO)
  2000 survey of health systems by, 23
  goals of, 24–25